MW01520675

OBESITY

Does it need a
Self-Balanced Lifestyle?

BY LEE B

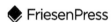 FriesenPress

One Printers Way
Altona, MB R0G 0B0
Canada

www.friesenpress.com

Copyright © 2024 by Lee B
First Edition — 2022

All rights reserved.

All rights reserved for this author's work to justify the accomplishment of the recommended requirements by the (2019-2020) University of Derby: Independent Scholarly Activity (ISA). Module code (7EL995/ assessment), UDOL-2019-09-23, which was completed and can be found on the following link: http://www.derby.ac.uk/research/ethics/policy-document.

Parts and materials contained in this book can be used in electronic retrieval for study reasons, personal purposes for therapeutic guidance, or statistical purposes only. No parts of this book can be copied or manipulated mechanically without the authorization of the author.

No part of this publication may be reproduced in any form, or by any means, electronic or mechanical, including photocopying, recording, or any information browsing, storage, or retrieval system, without permission in writing from FriesenPress.

ISBN
978-1-03-911390-9 (Hardcover)
978-1-03-911389-3 (Paperback)
978-1-03-911391-6 (eBook)
978-1-03-917773-4 (AudioBook)

1. MEDICAL, DISEASES
2. MEDICAL, RESEARCH
3. HEALTH & FITNESS, DISEASES

Distributed to the trade by The Ingram Book Company

OBESITY

PREFACE

This book is derived from the dissertation submitted to *The Postgraduate Program of the University of Derby* to complete the requirements for the degree in the *Master of Science* program.

The dissertation's title is: "How can Lifestyle Interventions Remedy Successfully the Self-Inflicted Canadian Obesity?"

This author's work explores the general causes of Overweight/Obesity and indicates that the individual can play an ultimate role to solve this condition.

Disclaimer: The material and illustrations displayed in this book are provided as they are according to their verifiable sources and accuracy. All information and materials are allowed to be used in any way by the public as needed in paper or any other type of work with regards to publications and tables, which are available on Statcan website,

https://www150.statcan.gc.ca/n1/pub/12-591-x/12-591-x2009001-eng.htm.

Consistent governmental sources have provided the materials for this thesis such as *The Public Health Agency of Canada* (*PHAC*), *Canadian Community Health Survey Data* (*CCHS*), as well as *Canadian Health Measures Survey* (*CHMS*).

ACKNOWLEDGMENT

This dissertation has been made possible with written published/secondary literature on obesity. The data has been obtained without any disturbance from consistent governmental sources such as *The Public Health Agency of Canada (PHAC), CCHS Data,* as well as *CHMS*.

All data has been gathered specifically from the Statcan website: https://www150. statcan.gc.ca/n1/pub/12-591-x/12-591-x2009001-eng.htm. High-quality data is available from different surveys as follow:

– Canadians' health and health habits.
– Trends in body mass index.
– Health fact sheets that supplied various data on health risk behaviors as well as health behavior scores.

I am very grateful for the accessibility of the information I gathered. For all, I express my sincere gratitude.

ABSTRACT

Recently, obesity rose worldwide at a sudden and fearful speed (Tran, 2014). Bray (2004) mentioned that obesity is induced by exorbitant energy, stowed as fat cells that intensify in quantity. These fat cells subsequently produce hyperplasia (enlargement of an organ by the multiplication of its cells' numbers) and hypertrophy (rise of the cells' size) (Bing.com, n.d.cd) which finally cause the pathology of obesity (Figure 10).

This study presents individual *lifestyle treatment interventions* (Jensen et al., 2013) as the most appropriate and successful procedure to remedy obesity.

Statistics Canada has been utilized, particularly the *CHMS* and the *CCHS* to trace and analyze:

1. Healthy Behaviors Scores (HBS),
2. The Body Mass Index (BMI),
3. The contrast of key Health Risk Behaviors (HRB) with obesity,
4. The correlation of HRB with obesity.

The statistical results show:

1. High physical inactivity among children and youth aged 5-17 years (Public Canada, 2017 & 2019).
2. High physical inactivity of adults aged 18 years and above (Public Canada, 2017, 2019; Statistics Canada, 2019f & 2020).
3. High sedentary behavior among children and youth in the last three years (Public Canada, 2017 & 2019).
4. Significant decrease in consumption of fruits and vegetables confirming an increase in unhealthy eating (Statistics Canada, 2015ab, 2017ab & 2019a).
5. Health Behavior Scores: only one or two provinces had an HBS above the national average rate (Statistics Canada, 2017c, 2017d & 2018a).
6. The obesity rate has tremendously increased from 17.9% (2009) to 26.8% (2018) (Statistics Canada, 2013, 2015defgh; 2018b & 2021b).

Finally, if an individual performs multiple HRB through their unhealthy life-style, they will subsequently become a causal agent of their overweight and obesity (123HelpMe.com., 2000-2018). The obesity epidemic involves the *self-inflicted character* (Obesitycanada.ca., 2019), which is linked to individual unhealthy behaviors (Halpern Bruno & Halpern Alfredo, 2014). Therefore, the appropriate remedy is the individual *lifestyle treatment interventions* (Bandura, 2005).

TABLE OF CONTENTS

TABLES

FIGURES AND IMAGES

CHAPTER 1

INTRODUCTION

Presently, the world is characterized by "Obesity soars to 'alarming' levels in developing countries" (Tran, 2014). From the beginning of 1985, Canada had a spectacular Intensification of its obesity rate by 200 percent (6.1 percent to 18.3 percent) (Twells et al., 2014 & 2008-2021), in relation with individual unhealthy lifestyle and obesogenic behaviors (Blaxter, 1990 & 123HelpMe.com., 2000-2018).

This unbelievable increase induced many associated diseases namely, "diabetes (type II), high blood pressure, atheromatosis, osteoarthrosis, sleep apnoea, depression, and damaged employment prospects" (GlobeNewswire News Room, 2019).

How can obesity and overweight be defined?

Both conditions are defined as atypical or extreme fat build-up in the body that could damage health (Who.int., 2021). Body mass index (BMI) has been considered as the individual's "weight in kilograms divided by the square meters of his height" (kg/m2) (Who.int., 2004).

Research has discovered the complex relationship between genetic and environmental factors that induce "adipocyte hypertrophy, hypoxia, a variety of stresses, and inflammatory processes within adipose tissue" (Blüher, 2009).

It is proven that obesity is linked to a pro-inflammatory disorder expressed by the enlargement of fat tissue, jointly with immune cells that promote the intensification of the quantity of *pro-inflammatory cytokines*. This phenomenon makes a cytokine storm (Figures B), which is a deregulated and extreme emission of *pro-inflammatory signaling molecules* (Asghar & Sheikh, 2017).

Another type of obesity is related to "*Melanocortin 4 receptor* (MC4R)", which involves mental delay, body deformation, and growth abnormality of certain organs (Huvenne et al., 2016). Also, obesity is induced by Prader-Willi Syndrome, which is a seldom genetic deficiency impacting almost one person out of 12, 000 individuals (Blackburn-Evans, 2004).

Beyond genetics, it was found that overweight and obesity are manifested by an *energy imbalance*, specifically, the "energy intake surpasses energy output", which induces a "low-grade, and long-lasting inflammation" (Johnson et al., 2012). Furthermore, obesity results from the build-up of "proinflammatory cells in visceral adipose tissue (VAT)" (Wensveen et al., 2015).

White fat stores energy in large greasy droplets all over the body, inducing obesity, while brown fat has reduced droplets and elevates quantities of mitochondria, which transforms fat into calories to power the body (Orlando, 2019).

Gordon-Larsen & Heymsfield (2018) have explained deeply obesity which can be conceptualized as an intricate, multi-factorial illness comprising of "genetic, biological, psychological, environmental, and socio-cultural factors". Amid these factors, impulsivity in obese individuals appears to have a special and significant role, Whiteside and Lynam (2001) have suggested four aspects of impulsivity that exist in obese individuals as follows: "Urgency, lack of premeditation, lack of perseverance, and sensation seeking." The cognitive and motivational functionalities associated with these four aspects of impulsivity can be investigated and described (Mobbs et al., 2007).

Figure 1: Obesity is a True Disease

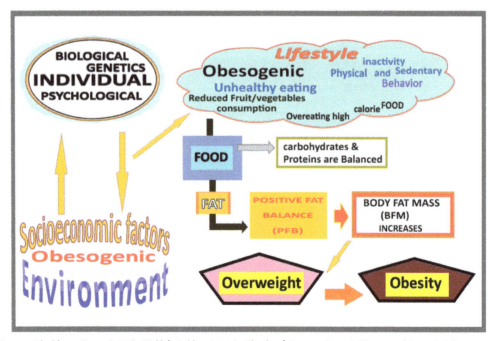

Source: *Blackburn-Evans (2004); Wolf & Colditz (1994); Elinder & Jansson (2008); Hammond (2009); Johnson et al. (2012); Lakerveld & Mackenbach (2017); Lev-Ran (2001); Neel (1962); Orlando (2019); Rosales (2018); Statistics Canada (2015ab; 2017ab & 2019a); Stigler et al. (2017); Venniyoor (2020); Who.int. (2004); Young (2018).*

This dissertation has a unique aim to critically analyze written, published/secondary literature on "obesity". Afterward, it will explore irrefutable facts of evidence confirming that obesity can be a "self-inflicted disease as it is considered in Canada" (Obesitycanada.ca., 2019). Furthermore, the dissertation will examine the *"self-initiated lifestyle strategies"*; then will explain how those strategies have the power to strongly induce the change of behavior to fight obesity by "regulating the motivation" (Bandura, 1998) and implementing "self-regulation skills" as well as "self-monitoring" diet and physical exercises (Bandura, 2005 & Jensen et al., 2013).

The specific objectives of this dissertation are to:

1. Define obesity: the mechanisms and pathophysiology (Figure 10); the link of metabolic syndrome to nutrition; the role of fat cells (white/brown). Establish evidence that every individual can be the causal agent of obesity: an individual's lifestyle behavior that increases weight and develops obesity.

2. Investigate how the individual becomes unable to lose weight and maintain reduced weight; the challenge of "overweight, diet, fast food, and physical exercises."

3. Explore the complexity of economic factors, socio-environmental factors (the role of obesogenic compounds in the development of obesity), and behavioral contributing factors that promote obesity such as a sedentary life.

4. Examine the relationship between overweight/obesity and mortality; the social stigma of obesity.

5. Critically examine the medical treatment effects, compare the medical to non-medical treatments and find the most appropriate management. Discuss how the same causal agent can apply self-initiated strategies to remedy obesity and finally, describe how self-initiated strategies work.

The rationale of this dissertation is to present individual *lifestyle treatment interventions* (Bandura, 2005 & Jensen et al., 2013) as the most appropriate and successful methods, strongly inducing the change of behavior to fight the *self-inflicted Canadian obesity* (Obesitycanada.ca., 2019 & GlobeNewswire News Room., 2019). This *self-inflicted obesity* is linked to several HRB (Public Canada, 2017) and this rationale is derived from the conclusion drawn from the results of statistical analysis of health indicators, specifically:

– Health Risk Behaviors contrasted with obesity shown in Table A.2 and Table A.3.
– Rise of physical inactivity of adults aged 18 years and above (Public Canada, 2017 & Statistics Canada, 2015fg).
– Rise of physical inactivity among children and youth from 5 to 17 years (Public Canada, 2017).
– Rise of sedentary behavior among children and youth in the last three years (Public Canada, 2017 & 2019).

This dissertation has seven chapters. Chapter 1 includes the definition of obesity regarding mechanisms, pathophysiology, the link of metabolic syndrome to nutrition, and the role of white and brown fat cells (Lee, 2016). Several pieces of evidence confirm that every individual can be the causal agent of obesity when the individual performs multiple risk behaviors in his lifestyle.

The body of an individual that carries an unhealthy lifestyle starts increasing weight and develops obesity (Figure 2).

These facts have been confirmed by the results of statistical analysis that are detailed and concluded in Chapter 4, including the relationship between mortality and the Pathology of Obesity (Figure 10) as well as the social stigma impact of obesity.

Chapter 2 is a Review of the Literature's section, which explores the complexity of obesity causes and the "Obesity Epidemic" that became a Canadian concern. Then, Chapter 2 also includes a summary of the existing literature on "how the individual becomes unable to lose weight and maintain reduced weight," as well as the challenge of "overweight, diet, fast food, and physical exercises."

Third, it explores the complexity of the *economic factors and socio-environmental factors* as well as the role of *obesogenic agents* in the development of obesity, and *behavioral contributing factors* that promote obesity such as sedentary life.

Chapter 3 is the methodology section that includes the description of the Case Study Design; also, the gathered data from Statistic Canada. Statistics Canada are the methods used to track and help critically analyze the trends in health behaviors and body mass of Canadians until 2018.

Key Health Risk Behaviors (HRB) have been "contrasted with medical conditions" and the "correlation of HRB" with "the medical condition of obesity" is explored as well.

Figure 2: Different intertwined Factors interact into the Genesis of Obesity

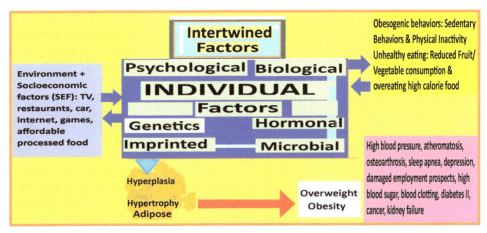

Source: Bing.com. (2007-2013); Bing.com. (n.d.a); Bing.com. (n.d.b); Bing.com. (n.d.c); Bing.com. (n.d.d); Darwish et al. (2020); Elinder & Jansson (2008); Fawcett & Barroso (2010); Gulati & Yeo (2013); Hammond (2009); Healthypeople.gov. (2014); Holtcamp (2012); Johnson et al. (2012); Lakerveld & Mackenbach (2017); Lukas et al. (1997); Mandal (2019); Who.int. (2004).

Chapter 4 discusses the Results of statistical analysis, which indicate the following:

1. Physical Inactivity among children and youth aged 5-17.

2. Adult Physical inactivity aged 18 years and above.

3. Sedentary Behavior among children and youth.

4. Fruit and vegetable consumption were conducted from 2013 to 2017.

5. Health Behavior Score were tracked during three or four consecutive years in all the Provinces from 2013, indicating the fluctuation of the proportion of scores higher versus lower but showing that many provinces having a lower HBS than the national average (NA).

6. The decrease in fruit and vegetable consumption. Finally, the statistical analysis indicates and demonstrates that obesity in Canada is induced by individual behaviors.

These behaviors can be performed by any individual and make the individual a potential *causal agent* of their overweight and obesity.

Chapter 5 discusses, reviews and reconsiders, in detail, diverse notions described namely the *self-inflicted character* of obesity in Canada, then points out the "individual as the causal agent" of their overweight and obesity.

The remedy needs to be the "*self-initiated lifestyle strategies*" which emerge from the statistical data tracked and analyzed in Chapter 4.

Chapter 6 includes Remedy's section on obesity which deeply examines the medical treatment effects, compares the medical to non-medical treatment. Then, the section analyses the failures and challenges faced by many medical approaches to battle obesity that have been found ineffective due to enormous resources devoted to disadvantageous health procedures. Furthermore, the pricey medical treatments fail to accomplish durable outcomes, after long-term therapies of recurrent disorders of obesity (Halpern Bruno & Halpern Alfredo, 2014), and discuss how the "same causal agent can apply self-initiated strategies" to remedy obesity. Then, it describes how *self-initiated strategies* work.

Chapter 7 summarizes the completion of the dissertation that describes the Lifestyle interventions that target *"individual health behaviors."*

CHAPTER 2

REVIEW OF LITERATURE

This chapter summarizes the current state of information concerning obesity as a complex disease, but a Canadian concern. This chronic health condition promotes several associated co-morbidities for the affected individuals and those who are potentially vulnerable to develop it, anywhere and at any time in Canada. Obesity became a foremost worldwide public health concern that particularly induces a variety of social and psychological debilities and various medical ailments namely "diabetes mellitus, gallbladder disease, osteoarthritis, heart disease, and some forms of cancer" (Bray, 2004).

In Canada, this challenge has required an urgent well-engineered intervention to avert its further expansion (Laws et al., 2014 & DiSalvo, 2017). This intervention (Figure 11) will perform the self-control, self-regulation, and self-monitoring of health behaviors (Bandura, 2005) displayed in Images 1, 2, 3, 4, and 5.

Image 1:
Physical Exercises

Image 2:
Eating Fruits and Vegetables

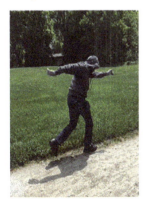

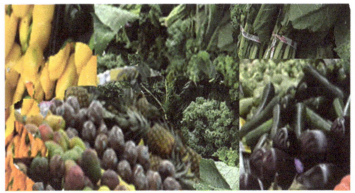

Source: (Banza, 2021a).

Source: (Banza, 2021b).

2.1 Introduction

The rate of the recurrent obesity phenomenon continues to rise during these current three decades with an extreme progression of Body Mass Index (BMI) rising from 35.0 to 39.9 and beyond 40.0. The rate of obesity that affects older individuals (18 years and above) in Canada has been amplified from 6.1 percent to 18.3 percent (Twells et al., 2014 & 2008-2021). Moreover, from 1985, the occurrence of classes I, II, and III rose from "5.1% to 13.1%"; while in 2019, the obesity rate in classes I was estimated to reach "14.8%, 4.4% for Class II and 2.0% for Class III". It was then projected that half of Canadians could be furthermore overweight and obese (adults 18 years and above) than "normal-weight adults" (Twells et al., 2014; 2008-2021).

It is obvious that, once an individual is informed about their obesity situation, their willingness and assurance is not sufficient to help them to correct their living conditions in order to reduce weight and sustain healthy average weight (Rosales, 2018). Obesity will remain a complex disease, but the individual will be the unique root cause of this phenomenon (123HelpMe.com., 2000-2018).

2.2 Complexity of Obesity Causes

The increase in the obesity rate in Canada became a very significant issue that requires a deep analysis of its causes. This phenomenon involves two aspects, namely the time of onset and the phases of intertwined (Figure 2) mechanisms comprising of "social and biological factors." Another analysis is required to explore the social and environmental factors (Figure 1) that promote obesity (Glass & McAtee, 2006).

Significant and possible intertwined factors at different stages have been found by evidence-based research as potential causes of obesity, explicitly:

- Genetic factors (Epstein et al., 2007).
- Neurobiology (DelParigi. et al., 2006) and psychological factors (Lindroos et al., 1997).
- Familial environment and various stressors (Seckl & Meaney, 2004).
- Social locations and social customs (Brewer et al., 1990).
- Built environment (Booth et al., 2005) as well as markets that have economic problems, their outcomes, and governmental/civic policy (Tillotson, 2004).

Several potential causes of obesity have been tested, also diverse pathways of obesity impacts have been examined, through various methodologies and departments of science that include "genetics, neuroscience, economics, and political science" (Hammond, 2009).

A study conducted by Zheng (2016) and other researchers found that obese individuals have:

– An elevated metabolic syndrome score.
– A rise of DNA methylation in the mitochondrial genes MT-CO1 and MT-ND6 and in the mitochondrion- related nuclear gene PPARGC1A.

Flaquer et al. (2014) found that "two mitochondrial single nucleotide polymorphisms (SNPs) located in the cytochrome c oxidase subunit genes (MT-CO1 and MT-CO3) and three mitochondrial SNPs located in the NADH dehydrogenase subunit genes (MT-ND1, MT-ND2, and MT-ND4L) were significantly associated with a higher BMI" (Stigler et al., 2017). A study conducted in 2007 found that "fat mass and obesity-associated protein (FTO)" was linked to adiposity; then, FTO functions as a regulator of eating attitudes and energy outflow (Fawcett & Barroso, 2010). The fat mass and obesity-associated protein were then linked to BMI increase and obesity (Gulati, & Yeo, 2013).

A series of diverse pathways function as inducers of obesity in the body, including the *individual-level factors,* which act on "dopamine-mediated reward and the mesocorticolimbic pathway" (Hammond, 2009). The "dopamine-4 (DRD4) and dopamine-2 (DRD2) receptors" have been found to stimulate the dopamine scheme and impact feeding and reward (Epstein et al., 2007).

The costs of obesity and its frequency across the globe are exorbitant and nothing indicates any sudden reduction, as Dr. Arya Sharma mentioned it, that the health care system has failed to correctly treat obesity; instead, the program has been treating the conditions that develop from obesity (Hrvatin, 2019). Obesity can be "easily treated by changing lifestyle, specifically changing unhealthy choices" (Katz, 2014). Moreover, obesity is considered as "complicated; so, as to be treated" (Tello, 2018).

Even if obesity (Figure 1) is considered a "complex, multi-factorial disease" with "genetic, behavioral, socioeconomic, and environmental origins" (Hruby & Hu, 2015) but it is strongly linked to individual behaviors (Katz, 2014; Sharma & Salas, 2018).

Ball and Crawford (2006) indicate that the relationship exists between socioeconomic functionality and obesity, which supports the explanation of the role of "social, physical, policy, and cultural environments (Figure 1)."

Currently, it is regrettable that available food that is rich in energy has an elevated sugar, fat, and salt composition and has been delivered in an eating environment that promotes food desires unrelated to the dietary recommendation, consequently increasing overweight and obesity (Birch, 1999). There is credible evidence that the increase in vegetables and fruit-eating could avert the rise of body mass (Boeing et al., 2012).

Research has found that neurobiological systems stimulate individual choices through decision-making when choosing food, and the dopamine-striatal structure system is influenced by such executive control (DelParigi et al., 2006).

Social standards and circumstances impact straightaway food feeding (De Castro et al., 1990) and indirectly impact the body image (Fitzgibbon et al., 2000). It is well documented that obesity is a sickness that propagates by social networks (Christakis & Fowler, 2007); by the facility to provide food, to get it in the nearby food retailers, restaurants, food preparation, schools, work, and at home, including the reduction of food price (Elinder & Jansson, 2008; Finkelstein et al., 2005).

It is also propagated by the "built environment" (Booth et al., 2005) and the complexity of "obesogenic economic and socio-environmental factors" that constitute the "markets and prices" (Hammond, 2009). Bray (2004) stated that obesity remains a long-lasting illness such as "hypertension and atherosclerosis". It has been established that obesity is the disproportion of energy intake (food) in comparison with the energy consumed.

The exorbitant energy is stowed as fat cells that intensify in quantity (Figure B). The pathology (Figure 10) of obesity is promoted by hyperplasia (enlargement of an organ by the cells' numbers that multiply) (Bing.com., n.d.c) and hypertrophy (rise of the cells' size) (Bing.com., n.d.d).

2.3   Obesity Epidemic became a Canadian Concern

Blackburn-Evans (2004) wrote about the unhealthy lifestyle carried by people and the rise of obesity which seriously concerned Doctor Berall who treats obese patients:

1. It swiftly began and progressively developed into a new lifestyle for future generations of all ages.

2. Obesity intensified in Canada and worldwide.

3. The World Health Organization (Who.int., 2004) has officially considered "obesity as an epidemic disease" because of the multiplicity of ailments that are linked to it.

4. Scientists are laboring hard to understand and tackle the complexity of sicknesses linked to obesity.

Canadians are so larger than a generation ago, and the question to ask is why this is currently happening?

The Canadian Population Health Initiative described that during the last twenty years, overweight and obesity triplicated for children and folded for adults (Blackburn-Evans, 2004). Several individuals continue living a sedentary life, which induces the present obesity epidemic as a result of a combined obesogenic environment and exorbitant food consumption along with physical inactivity (Who.int., 2004).

Anderson (2004b) acknowledged that "our changing environment" is mostly responsible for inducing obesity, as this environment has more available and cheaper food that is served in larger quantities with frequent snacking which supply high and quick excess of calories as nourishment concerns (Blackburn-Evans, 2004).

Penfold (2004 – 2011) acknowledged that the *"car-induced expansion"* has created a *"suburban Canada's dependence on the automobile"; this car dependency* was found as an increasing obesity factor that raises it to 3% when the individual is seated in the car for 30 minutes while it is being driven (Holmes, 2022).

The social life of Canadians relies on driving cars to socialize, work, reach their place of work, enjoy leisure, entertain in the parks, travel to other provinces, and accomplish many businesses anywhere at any time (Blackburn-Evans, 2004).

The World Health Organization (WHO) stated that the ultimate sources of the *Obesity Epidemic* are societal, which are induced by the environment that encourages sedentary lifestyles and food intake rich in fat (Who.int., 2004). A daily reduction of energy outflow can induce obesity when the individual reduces physical activities (Hill et al., 2000).

Often, obese individuals can be impelled to tumble into an infighting emotional circle associated with different psychological manifestations such as "anger, sadness, excitement", and exaggerated hunger, and food as a unique "exit for those feelings" (Rosales, 2018).

Several drugs induce overweight and obesity (Table A.1) such as "antidepressants, anticonvulsants or anti-epileptics and corticosteroids" (Ben-Menachem, 2007; Cheng & Kashyap, 2010; Apovian et al., 2015 as adopted by Heymsfield et al., 2018; Rosales, 2018).

Blackburn-Evans (2004) quoted the word of Anderson (2004a) which stated that "our changing environment is largely to blame as the cause of obesity in Canada"; when the environmental factors inter-mix with our social and individual characteristics, specifically "age, gender, socioeconomic status, race, education level, ethnicity, and disability status", they altogether impact diet and physical movements (Healthypeople.gov., 2014).

Sobal (2001) mentioned that the introduction of Western food systems such as technological advances in food processing, transportation, affordability, and limitless quantities of quite low-priced foods in grocery stores, cookery, retailing, and ready-made. Adding to this situation are "home-delivered, drive through, and fast/snack foods" that have contributed to the *Obesity Epidemic*.

One occurrence where genetic induce obesity is the occasional Prader-Willi illness, which is a genetic sickness affecting approximately one individual in 12,000. This occurrence links several disorders to Prader, particularly obesity and excess appetite which makes the brain incapable of identifying the complete signals stimulus (Blackburn-Evans, 2004).

Every year an individual increases by two pounds of weight, and beyond 35 years an individual might become overweight as they become older; also research demonstrated that the lack of sleep stimulates the exaggerated hunger for high-calorie index food (Rosales, 2018).

Sleep deprivation causes a deregulation of hormonal functions in human which stimulates the "overeating and weight gain". Sleep shortage changes the making and the functioning of "Leptin and ghrelin hormones" which normally regulate the appetite. Sleep shortage induces the insufficiency of growth hormone which in turn increases cortisol hormone production, then deregulate the "metabolism of food" which finally causes obesity (Rehman, 2023).

Adiposity as well as increased weight in obesity have mechanical impacts on digestive apparatus "esophagus" , and cause linked-metabolic conditions comprising of "insulin resistance, hypertension, and dyslipidemia" (Nam, 2017).

The incidence of "obesity can be promoted by the built environment" when it lacks shops to supply fruit and vegetables, and lacks safe, accessible, and motivational areas to play or to exercise physically (Healthypeople.gov., 2014).

The culture of relying on cars has induced the story of juvenile obesity; when transporting children to school for reasons of safety or when hurrying to not be late. This condition truly reduced individual possibilities of walking (Blackburn-Evans, 2004).

Kaplan (1992) stated that physical exercise (Image 1) and a balanced diet carried by people of every age and socioeconomic status have been acknowledged as a fundamental key to sustaining a healthy lifestyle. Convincing evidence shows the existence of "relationships between physical activity, lifestyle, and health" (Lukas et al., 1997).

However, genes can induce obesity through "positive energy balance over time" which accumulates calories in the body to accomplish that potential phenomenon (Lev-Ran, 2001).

Some daily activities can promote obesity specifically: the lack of satisfactory physical exercises whether individual or public (costly) or elongated times of working in a sitting position with reduced time to exercise; then, poor inactivity combines with multiples advertisements that promote the consumption of a large quantity of food in restaurants, almost every article around individuals promote consciously or unconsciously the increase of weight (Rosales, 2018).

Several Indigenous Peoples living in Canada have strong *gene-environment interaction* called the *thrifty gene* hypothesis (Neel, 1962).

The hypothesis stipulates that individuals grow robust biological functionalities to preserve energy; precisely fat that allows them to subsist during famine periods. Nowadays, people have an abundance of food, and the *thrifty genes* induce obesity due to the quick social changes, which can be explained as a phenomenon that started from "*the distant past, as these genes helped the organism to improve energy efficiency and store excess energy safely as fat to survive periods of famine, but in the present day obesogenic environment, have turned them detrimental*" (Venniyoor, 2020). Researchers have indicated that there was link "between high birth-weight and diabetes" Among Aboriginals (Dyck et al., 2001). Since the "Neel's thrifty genes" was solely related to "Diabetes Mellitus 2"; the hypothesis stretched to include specifically "obesity" (Neel, 1962).

Generally, obese individuals—particularly binge eaters—are susceptible to become much impulsive in comparison with thin individuals. Several impulsive individuals have reduced control over-eating behavior, subsequently, impulsivity has been linked to overweight all of the time according to research (Nederkoorn et al., 2007).

2.4 Some Lifestyle Activities in Canada Relate to the Prevalence of Obesity

The daily physical inactivity promotes obesity when it is linked to different activities such as the "dependency on the automobile", a study led by "Lawrence D. Frank, PhD" found that just 30 minutes spent by a seated individual in a driven car increases 3% of his weight which could lead to obesity (Holmes, 2022). Tomalty & Mallach (2009) estimated the relationship between the *"community design factors such as land use, street connectivity, sidewalks"* with *walking and biking activity*, and their impacts on health, then their study indicated that there is much relationship between enhanced walkability and additional walking and cycling activity, to reduce the *"body mass index (BMI), and lower hypertension."*

The Canadian environment accumulates an extra load of multiple obesogenic factors, together with the way individuals handle their stress and cope with the impacts of the obesogenic environment in their daily life (Rosales, 2018).

The HBS in Canada are evaluated by the following health indicators (Statistics Canada, 2017d):
– The consumption of fruits and vegetables.
– Heavy drinking, smoking and
– Physical activity.

Sedentary behaviors of children are related to the fast change of technology, as well as the amplification of internet utilization, and social network-popularity (Public Canada, 2017). It has been established that city development promotes obesity due to the associations of walkability and "obesity, type 2 diabetes, and hypertension" (Colley et al., 2019).

The Canadian experience indicates that Canadians are stressed. Stress is one cause of obesity. Stress in Canada is induced in different ways (Statistics Canada, 2015c):
1. One out of four people in Canada accuses stress to be the reason for leaving their job.
2. Seventy-three workers in Canada, between ages 20 to 64, mentioned having stress.
3. Twenty-three percent of Canadians aged 15 years and older mentioned having everyday stress and also stated that each day they are tremendously worried.

4. Thus far, the proportion of stressed individuals rose to 30% in adults between ages 35 to 54; subsequently causing "mental health problems, work absenteeism, finances struggles, and new modern concerns."

Canada ranks amongst the worst countries in the "Organization for Economic Cooperation and Development" and has a high rate of adult obesity (Public Canada, 2017).

Obesity in Canada is linked to attitudes taken by each individual than to a hereditarily programmed condition (Rosales, 2018). Friedman (2015) stated that: *Living a sedentary lifestyle is a major risk factor for obesity and diabetes. He believes that planning and building communities that promote physical activity will help to reduce the occurrence of those diseases, cities and homes have to be exercise machines that help people living there to be less prone to obesity and diabetes*" (Www.CBC News.ca., 2015).

2.5   Obesity's Self-Inflicted Character is an Individual Factor

One issue publicized in the "2017 Report Card," mentions that "obesity in Canada is not recognized" as a "chronic disease by the federal government or any provincial/territorial governments." Though obesity was recognized by "the Canadian Medical Association's and the medical professional associations in Saskatchewan and Yukon."

Obesity remains a disease, so far, without any official guidelines or policies set to remedy or manage it in any province and territory.

Being a self-inflicted risk factor, obesity negatively impacts strategies and intervention measures undertaken by the Ministry of Health in Canada (Obesitycanada.ca., 2019). The etiology of obesity can be conceptualized as follows:

1. The Individual-Level Factors (Figure 3) are located in the distant upstream region that comprises of "biological, genetic, and psychological influencing components such as knowledge, motivation, and the ability to manipulate the upstream obesogenic behaviors. "

Figure 3: Individual-Level Factors

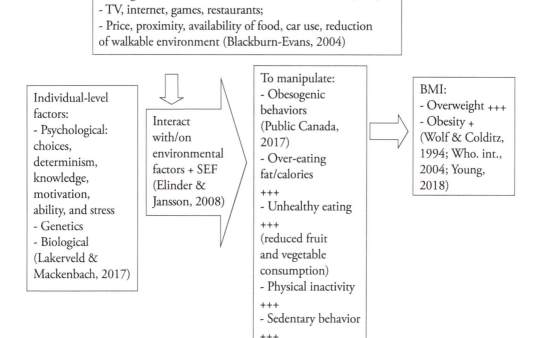

Source: Blackburn-Evans (2004); Elinder & Jansson (2008); Lakerveld & Mackenbach (2017); Public Canada (2017); Wolf & Colditz (1994); Who.int. (2004); Young (2018).

2. Following psychological factors such as "choices, determinations, motivations, stress, lack of sleeping, and impulsivity" act in concert with other metabolic factors to activate and stimulate other pathways that cause fat cells inflammation with different strengths, daily, yearly, or during the lifespan.

3. They act through environmental and socioeconomic factors (food price, availability, preferences, screen time).

4. They influence or manipulate different health behaviors (eating, sedentary behavior, physical inactivity) and finally increase overweight and obesity (Lakerveld & Mackenbach, 2017).

Though the onset of obesity remains very complex in Canada, the physiology of obesity begins in the individual with the lack of equilibrium between calories supplied from food eaten and calories disbursed (Who.int., 2021).

This onset is associated with the following activities:

a. Physical inactivity (Public Canada, 2017).

b. Sleep shortage (Patel and Hu, 2008).

c. Amplification of stress (Block et al., 2009).

d. Lower motivation and reduced intensity of self-initiated physical exercise and high sedentary activities, particularly extended time watching television or gaming which relate to the increase of risk of "obesity and type 2 diabetes", while low to modest activity reduce these health issues (Hu et al., 2003).

e. The increase of technology, specifically internet development and other sedentary activities, has substantially reduced physical movement and increased unhealthy behaviors that promote further obesity (Kaplan, 1992).

The weight of fat will accumulate and then cause a series of symptoms, particularly:

a. Sleep apnea and osteoarthritis by compressing the throat or wearing and tearing the joints.

b. The metabolic influences of inflamed fat cells can affect at distance or can induce the release of particular chemicals, such as "free fatty acids and several peptides" that might compress the surrounding tissues by their extra weight or intensify the secretion of inflammatory chemicals (Bray, 2004).

In most cases, as shown in Figure B, the immune cells are responsible for "obesity-induced adipose tissue inflammation" (Wensveen et al., 2015; Byung-Cheol & Jongsoon, 2013). These inflamed fat cells (Figure B) are in a state of "hyperplasia, hypertrophy or both which are combined to immune cells" that promote the secretion of "pro-inflammatory cytokines" causing "low-grade chronic inflammation in obesity" (Bing.com., n.d.cd). Inherited reduction of creatine metabolism in fat cells obstructs the "diet-induced thermogenesis" and induces obesity as well (Kazak et al., 2017).

However, the individual-level factors, namely lifestyle choices (Halpern Bruno & Halpern Alfredo, 2014; Sanders, 2017; Katz, 2014) incite individuals to carry unhealthy behaviors such as engaging in heavy drinking of alcohol, smoking, reduced eating of fruit and vegetables, or not performing physical activity and carrying sedentary lifestyle (GlobeNewswire News Room, 2019; Obesitycanada.ca., 2019; Public Canada, 2017).

These conditions subsequently make the individual a *causal agent* of their overweight and obesity (123HelpMe.com., 2000-2018). The individual becomes unable to lose weight and maintain reduced weight, due to powerful unhealthy influences that dictate their decisions to carry a poor lifestyle, being promoted by cheaper unhealthy food that is available at home, in restaurants, as well as in the convenience shops (Elinder & Jansson, 2008).

Diverse characteristics of psychological well-being such as body image is also manipulated by obesogenic behaviors namely, "sedentary behavior, physical activity, and diet" (Huang et al., 2007, Finne et al., 2013). Undeniably, media, family, peers, and social influences can impact the body image of any person, especially youth. Body image is fashioned through "environment, physical sensations, emotions, and physical experience" (Croll, 2005). The obese individual can have feelings of stigmatization created by their body image; a feeling of "great disapproval" (Www.thefreedictionary.com., 2003-2020) which reduces efforts to find the appropriate solution to the condition.

A study was conducted on the ability to address the negative feelings about Body Image (BI) specifically decreasing "body shame and disembodiment" and stimulating "positive BI" (by intensifying self-compassion and positive embodiment) (Burychka et al., 2021).

The 1960s economic development brought a supply and demand system that dramatically changed and increased a wide-reaching capability of the way food supply became organized and delivered. Then, it increased access to the surrounding stores of food and retailers' shops (White, 2007). Such factors brought the "over-consumption of high-energy foods and a lack of physical activity," which progressively induced overweight and obesity (Heymsfield & Wadden, 2017). Many countries, including Canada, promoted reliance on cars and residents became car-dependent to travel in the cities.

This condition endangered the environmental and socioeconomic well-being of individuals living in Canadian towns. The land use and transportation circumstances were transformed and developed into towns that rely on motor vehicles; subsequently, the residents had reduced biking and walking options for urban travel. Research indicates that individuals who walk from one place to another weigh typically seven pounds fewer than those who drive in the car (Chai, 2015).

Why aren't all Canadians Obese at the same time?

Several Canadians carry a similar lifestyle, full of obesogenic conditions that can predispose them to develop obesity during their lifetime, but not every Canadian becomes obese despite the obesogenic environment that surrounds them (Elinder & Jansson, 2008). Obesity is caused by individual unhealthy behaviors that relate them to the *self-inflicted character*; this why all Canadians are not obese at the same time (123HelpMe.com., 2000-2018).

Many Canadians miss going to sleep at night because they spend their nights watching movies and playing games, which creates unhealthy choices ending with an increase in weight. Currently, individuals are propelled down the road to unhealthy eating choices under any circumstance. Nevertheless, unhealthy eating spreads over a lifetime, not a single portion of festivity and activity remained unaffected.

People are compelled to allow themselves the enjoyment of a certain pleasure and eat large quantity of food during these functions; constantly continuing living in an environment that inclines them, and living in a condition with little chance of moving away from an unhealthy lifestyle (Young, 2018 & kazak, 2017).

Thus, the appropriate treatment can be initiated and implemented by the same individual who is the *causal agent* of their obesity through lifestyle intervention treatment (Jensen et al., 2013; Bandura, 1998- 2005).

Figure 4: Percentage of Obesity; Millions of Obese Persons Versus the Canadian Population

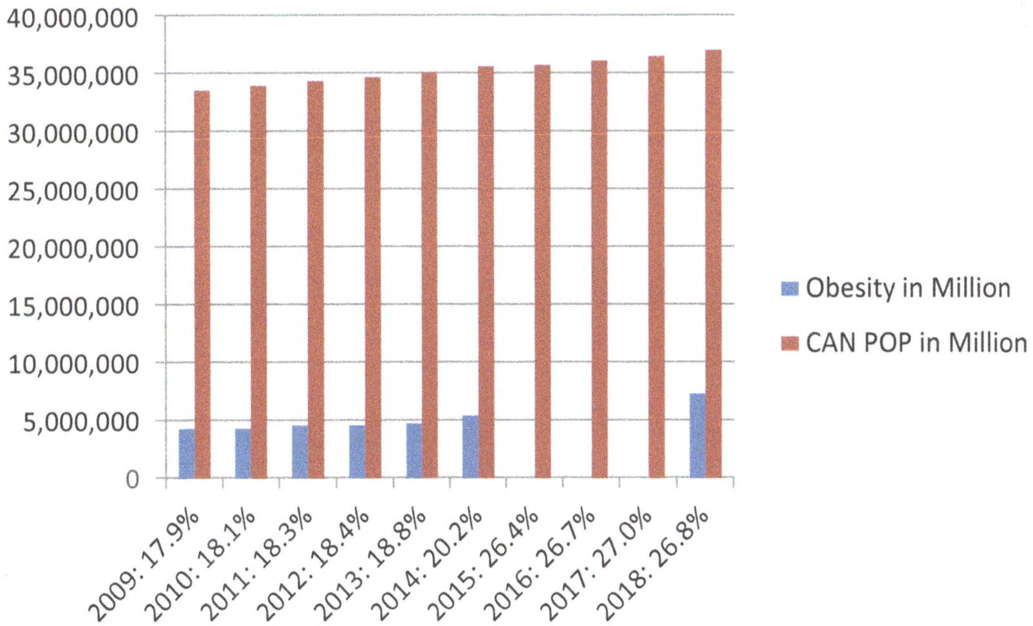

Source: Statistics Canada (2013, 2015defgh, 2018b & 2019e, 2021ab).

2.6 Summary

Obesity has been documented as a disease caused by multiple and complex factors such as the contextual aspects associated with "dwellings, educational facilities, nearby conditions", and the unhealthy lifestyle carried by an individual (Affenito et al., 2012).

This dissertation emphasizes individual behaviors as primary factors that induce obesity in Canada, namely diet, physical activity, and a sedentary lifestyle will be analyzed in the following chapters related to the analysis of health indicators.

General literature documents the multifaceted causes of obesity, which needs to include the root cause of this disease in order to deal with it successfully. In the definition of the root cause of obesity, this gap has persisted for a long period.

Thorough research has come to find that the onset of obesity is linked to individual lifestyle behavior after decades of consecutive surveys, such as the *CHMS* (Statistics Canada., 2019a) and *CCHS* (Statistics Canada., 2019b).

These different surveys conducted by both the *CHMS* and *CCHS* have established that obesity in Canada is primarily related to individual obesogenic behaviors.

Image 3: Sedentary Lifestyle

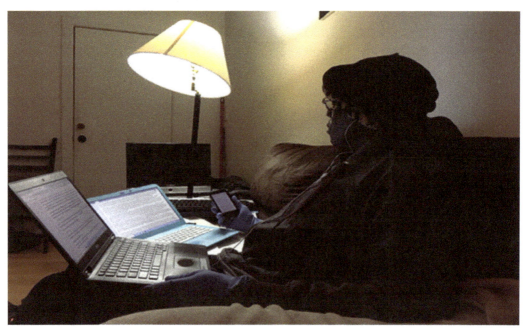

Source: (Banza, 2021c).

Available and updated information on Canadian obesity gave documented and detailed results that confirm the association of the disease with the *self-inflicted character* that promotes the *obesity epidemic fear*.

As an illustration, let's say that Mr. John is a 37-year-old, single man who lives in a suburb situated eight kilometers away from his workplace. Mr. John lives in an obesogenic environment (Image 3) which incites him to perform unhealthy behaviors such as sleeping very few hours while watching television during the night and playing different games on the computer.

He eats fast food rich in proteins, sugar, and fat that are delivered directly to his home. He consumes rarely fruits and vegetables. He drinks strong alcohol and smokes a packet of cigarettes every day. When he wakes up, he uses his car to go to work (Image 4) and works long hours in a sitting position. He sleeps only few hours during the night. He lacks time to walk and to exercise physically. After living this kind of life for a long period, he notices that his weight has tremendously increased and he becomes obese.

This individual lived an unhealthy lifestyle which made him obese (Public Canada, 2017). This individual will continue failing to lose his weight and maintain any reduced weight as long as he continues performing such unhealthy behaviors.

He will fail to balance his diet while fast food will be the first choice (Image 5) that attracts him, and his car will not allow him to walk. His work will not help him in any way to exercise physically. Mr. John will be enclosed in a system that gives him little hope to improve his lifestyle; subsequently, obesity will be the last lifestyle he might live for the rest of his life (Blackburn-Evans, 2004).

Mr. John chose to live this kind of life.

Can genes or metabolic disorders be responsible for his obesity?

If not, how did Mr. John become obese?

In the following chapter, health indicators will be sufficiently analyzed and will indicate the role of unhealthy behaviors that induced the obesity of Mr. John, as it has been described in the story above. Individual life cycle is directed by *free Healthy Choices versus free Unhealthy Choices*, anyone can be a Potential Healer/Fighter or a Potential Promoter of Overweight and Obesity (FUCIL) (Figure 5).

Figure 5: Free Unhealthy Choices Insecure Life (FUCIL)

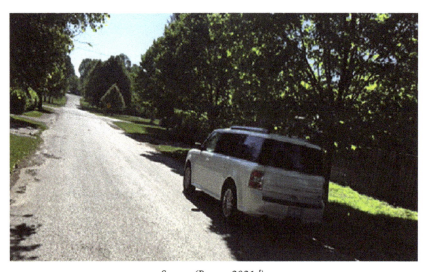

Individual life cycle is directed by free healthy choices vs. free unhealthy choices

Anyone can be a Potential Fighter/ Healer of Overweight and Obesity

Anyone can be a Potential Promoter of Overweight and Obesity

Whoever performs multiple obesogenic activities:
-Reducing the consumption of Fruits and vegetables
-Increasing Physical inactivity and sedentary lifestyle
-Overeating high calorie FOOD
-Live in conditions that deprive or reduce good quality of sleep
Being exposed to stressful activities

Free Unhealthy Choices Insecure Life

Lee B

Lifestyle Treatment
Fix Goals & Plan
To Self-control, Self-manage, Be-Self determined and Be-motivated to Self-regulate & Self-monitor:
-Weight/Diet
-Physical/Sedentary activities and Increase eating Fruit/vegetables

Overweight +++
Obesity +
Complications +

Source: Bandura (1997; 1998; 2005); Chai & Tang (2017); Colley et al. (2019); DelParigi et al. (2006); Elinder & Jansson (2008); Halpern Bruno & Halpern Alfredo (2014); Jensen et al. (2013); Kang & Park (2012); Katz (2014); Kong et al. (2020); Lakerveld et al. (2015); MacLean et al. (2015); Obesitycanada.ca. (2019); Public Canada (2017); Sanders (2017); Study.com. (2003); Tello (2017); Who.int. (2004).

Image 4: Individuals Drive Cars (Have reduced Physical Exercises)

Source: (Banza, 2021d).

Table 1: Percentage of Obesity; Millions of Obese Persons Versus the Canadian Population

Years/Percentage of Obesity	Obesity in Million	CAN POP in Million
2009: 17.9%	4,400,000	33,628,895
2010: 18.1%	4,500,000	34,004,889
2011: 18.3%	4,600,000	34,339,328
2012: 18.4%	4,700,000	34,714,222
2013: 18.8%	4,900,000	35,082,954
2014: 20.2%	5,300,000	35,437,435
2015: 26.4%	-	35,702,908
2016: 26.7%	-	36,109,487
2017: 27.0%	-	36,545,236
2018: 26.8%	7,300,000	37,065,084

Source: Statistics Canada (2013, 2015defgh, 2018b & 2019e, 2021ab).

Image 5: Processed Food

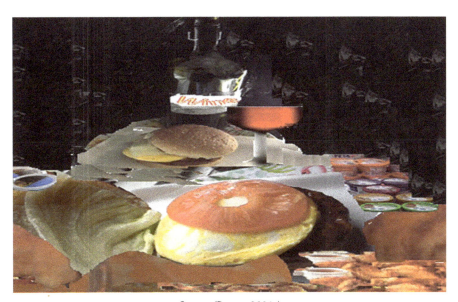

Source: (Banza, 2021e).

CHAPTER 3

METHODOLOGY

3.1   Case Study Design

This dissertation is a case study (Meijden et al., 2003) that uses the descriptive research design (Acasestudy.com., n.d.; Borg & Gall, 1989). It specifically explores data obtained from Statistics Canada sources, namely the *CHMS* and *CCHS*. This dissertation critically analyzes the results of statistics collected from health indicators of Canadians and links individual behaviors to the prevalence of obesity in Canada. The most matching treatment will derive from that link which will consist of health education through *lifestyle interventions* (Bandura, 2005; Jensen et al., 2013).

Such a selected approach is a suitable methodology to analyze the ongoing complexity of obesity (Acasestudy.com, n.d.) in Canada. The case study explores, investigates, and analyzes various pieces of evidence that show that obesity in Canada is a *self-inflicted disease* (GlobeNewswire News Room., 2019; Obesitycanada.ca., 2019). Several recent and published Statistics Canada sources are the main tools for this analysis.

3.2   Methods

This study uses the following Statistics Canada information, namely:

The *CHMS*, utilized since 2007 as means to gather information linked to the health of Canadians through conducted questions consisting of a household interview, as well as performing medical tests that include individuals invited to a *mobile examination center* for specific tests of vision tests, blood pressure, bone density, height, and weight (Statistics Canada, 2019c).

This study also focuses on collected *CHMS* measurements related to individual risk behaviors, specifically HBS that include healthy eating (nutrition), smoking behaviors, heavy drinking (alcohol), sedentary behaviors, and physical inactivity (fitness) (Public

Canada, 2017). The BMI of Canadians is traced through *CHMS* to "assess the prevalence of obesity in Canada" (Burton et al., 1985).

The *CCHS* has been efficient in the "health surveillance of the population and research" (Statistics Canada, 2019d) and carefully chosen indicators have been explored in these surveys such as the eating habits in comparison with the socio-demographic characteristics of individuals (age, sex, household income, and Aboriginal status) (Roblin et al., 2017). These surveys will help to trace obesity in Canada and link them to different HRB, namely physical inactivity, unhealthy eating (fruit and vegetable consumption); sedentary behavior, and HBS (Table 3).

The analysis of the "trends in the incidence of overweight and obesity" reflect the variation of reported or measured (BMI) of individuals and the analysis of HBSs as reported by the *PHAC* for a period of 10 to 15 years (Public Canada, 2017).

The broad worldwide literature on obesity details various determinants of obesity and obesogenic environments. The used methods to conduct this study target the "role of the individual and his lifestyle behaviors," particularly "unhealthy diet, physical inactivity" (Who.int., 2004) and "sedentary behaviors" (Heinonen et al., 2013).

3.3   Critical Tracking and Analysis of Trends in Health Behaviors and Body Mass

- A.1: Healthy Behaviors Scores
- A.2: Body Mass Index
- B: Key Health Risk Behaviors Contrasted with Medical Conditions
- C: Correlation of Health Risk Behaviors with the Medical Condition of Obesity

3.3. A.1   Health Risk Behaviors

The analysis of the failure to meet healthy living norms will confirm evidently that every individual can potentially be the causal agent of his or her obesity. Undoubtedly, the deep examination of individual lifestyle carried with excessive multiple HRBs (Public Canada, 2017) ascertains that the *self-inflicted obesity character* (GlobeNewswire News Room., 2019; Obesitycanada.ca., 2019) is subsequently induced by the individual's unhealthy lifestyle (Halpern Bruno & Halpern Alfredo, 2014; Sanders, 2017; Katz, 2014). These individual *decisions and behaviors* are achieved through the "social, physical, and economic environments" of the working, learning, and daily living (Public Canada, 2017).

3.3. A.1.1   Physical Activities, Fruit and Vegetable Consumed, and HBS

The healthy living indicators are represented in percentage, namely the level of physical inactivity of Canadian individuals 12 years and above; the "sedentary behaviors of kids in relation with the quick change of technology, the amplification of internet utilization, and social network-popularity" (Public Canada, 2017) and the "fruit and vegetable consumption" of individuals aged 12 years and above (Statistics Canada, 2017ab; 2019a).

3.3. A.1.2   The Physical Activity Survey

The surveys conducted on physical activity during the period of 2009 and 2011 *CHMS* show that "49.6% of children/youth aged 5 to 17 years" failed to satisfy the requirements of the *Canadian Sedentary Behavior Guidelines* (Public Canada, 2017).

Physical inactivity is recognized as a significant public health worry for individuals in Canada. The World Health Organization has recognized it as "the fourth leading risk factor for global mortality" and related it to several long-lasting illnesses, comprising of "cancer, cardiovascular diseases, and diabetes" (Apps.who.int., 2010).

The *CHMS* conducted during 2012 and 2013 indicated that 77.8% (20.1 million) individuals 18 years and over, and 90.7% of children/youth failed to satisfy the requirements of the *Canadian Physical Activity Guidelines* (*PAG*). Such surveys conducted on children/youth aged 5 to 17 years during the same period indicate that 51.8% of this group's age failed to satisfy the requirements of the *Canadian Sedentary Behavior Guidelines* (*SBG*) (Public Canada, 2017).

The 2014-2015 *CHMS* indicated that only 17.5% of individuals 18 years and above reached the *PAG* in completing more or less "150 minutes of moderate-to-vigorous physical activity each week, in bouts of 10 minutes." This indication means that 82.5% failed to meet the expectation (Public Canada, 2019).

The 2014-2015 *CHMS* related to screen-based sedentary behaviors and indicated that only 28.5% of children and youth met the recommendation of seating during two hours in front of a screen watching television/working on the computer, playing games during their leisure time; also, 37.6 % of children and youth met the recommended *PAG* (Public Canada, 2019).

According to the 2015 and 2016 *CHMS*, participants stated that they completed 49 minutes of physical activity every day; while the "physical activity measured by accelerometer" showed that they have only completed 23 minutes (Abedi, 2018). Also, the 2016 and 2017 *CHMS* on physical activity indicated that "only about 40% of children/youth" have satisfied the *PAG* while 60% failed to meet the expected requirement (Statistics Canada, 2019b).

The 2016 and 2017 *CHMS* mentioned that 16.4% of adults (*18 years and above*) satisfied the expected *Canadian 24-Hour Movement Guidelines* (Statistics Canada, 2019f).

In 2017, *12 year-olds* and above achieved 57.4% of *PAG*; *18-year-olds to 34* achieved 68.1%; *35-year-olds to 49* achieved 60.4%; *50-year-olds to 64* achieved 56.2%; and *65-year-olds and above* achieved only 40.6%, which was below the recommended *PAG* of 50% (Statistics Canada, 2020).

In 2018, *12 year-olds and above* achieved 54.6% of *PAG*; *18-year-olds to 34* achieved 64.3%; *35-year-olds to 49* achieved 58.4%; *50-year-olds to 64* achieved 54.0%; and *65 years old and above* achieved only 37.3%, which was below the recommended *PAG* (Statistics Canada, 2020). In 2016 and 2017, approximately 40% of children aged 5 years to 17 reached the expected activity requirement (Statistics Canada, 2019f).

3.3. A.1.3   Fruit and Vegetable Consumption Surveys

The following surveys were conducted with individuals aged 12 years and above living in Canada "who reported having consumed five or more times per day":
- The 2013 *CCHS* stated that 40.8% of individuals aged *12 and older* living in Canada, approximately 11.5 million, reached the NA. Only Quebec had 46.9%, which was above the national average (NA), and eight provinces had a lower rate that failed to reach the NA of 40.8% (Statistics Canada, 2015a).
- The 2014 *CCHS* indicated that 39.5% of approximately 11.2 million individuals aged *12 and over* living in Canada reached the NA (*consumed fruit and vegetables five or more times per day*). Only Quebec had 46.3%, which was above the NA rate of 39.5%, nine provinces had a lower rate than the NA rate (Statistics Canada, 2015b).

– The 2015 *CCHS* indicated that 31.5% of individuals aged *12 and older* living in Canada, nearly 9 million individuals, reached the NA, five provinces had a lower rate than the NA of 31.5%, and only Quebec had 38.8%, which was a higher rate than the NA (Statistics Canada, 2017a).

– The 2016 *CCHS* indicated that 30.0% of individuals aged *12 and older* in Canada, approximately 8.6 million individuals, reached the NA. Quebec had the highest percentage of 38.4%, less than 1 in 5 (18.3%) in Newfoundland and Labrador stated to consume five or more times everyday fruit/ vegetable (Statistics Canada, 2017b).

– The 2017 *CCHS* indicated that 28.6% of individuals aged *12 and older* living in Canada, approximately 8.3 million individuals, reached the NA. Research indicated that higher sedentary behavior was linked to "unhealthy dietary behaviors." The number of persons who stated to have consumed fruits and vegetables several times more than five has reduced, while the time of those who watched TV/games in a sitting position has increased (Statistics Canada, 2019a).

3.3. A.1.4   Healthy Behavior Scores

These surveys were conducted with individuals aged 18 years and above living in Canada. The Health Behavior Scores (HBS) of 3 or 4 is a combined score in a single one that indicates the wealth of healthy behaviors a person has to complete such as smoking, drinking alcohol, eating fruit/ vegetable, and exercising physically:

– In 2015, the *CCHS* indicated that 50.9% of individuals aged *18 and above* living in Canada, approximately 13.2 million, reached the expected HBS of 3 or 4; two provinces had an HBS above the NA of 50.9 %, namely Alberta at 53% and British Columbia at 57.3%; six provinces had a lower score rate than the NA, while Prince Edward Island and Quebec had a similar rate to the NA (Statistics Canada, 2017c).

– In 2016, the *CCHS* has indicated that 51.5% of individuals aged *18 and above* living in Canada, approximately 13.5 million individuals, had an HBS of 3 or 4, while British Columbia had the highest rate of 60% above the NA (51.5%). Five provinces had a lower score than the NA (Statistics Canada, 2017d).

– In 2017, the *CCHS* mentioned that 50.4% of individuals living in Canada *18 years and above*, approximately 13.4 million individuals reached the HBS of 3 or

4; British Columbia had the highest rate of 56.1% than the NA (50.4%); four provinces had a lower rate than the NA (Statistics Canada, 2018a).

3.3. A.2 The Body Mass Index

The frequency of obesity in Canada has been assessed by measuring the BMI, once established and recommended by the 1985 "National Institutes of Health (NIH) as a standard to evaluate individual patients for overweight and obesity" (Sanders, 2017).

The BMI of overweight and obese individuals are tracked (Public Canada, 2017) along with a critical examination of the:

- Trend analysis of BMI prevalence from 1985 to 2011 (Twells et al., 2014).
- Trend analysis of BMI "predictions of future prevalence" from 2013 to 2019 (Twells et al., 2008-2021).

A gradual rise in overweight and obesity occurred in 13 years. The following data relates to five consecutive years: the obesity rate was 5.6% in 1985; 9.2% in 1990; 13.4% in 1994; 12.7% in 1996, and 14.8% in 1998, while the population was only estimated at 22.2 million (Statistics Canada, 2001: *Annual demographic statistics, 2000.* Ottawa: Cat no 91-213-XPB) as reported by Katzmarzyk (2002b). The overweight and obesity in men rose from 47.0% during the period of 1970 to 1972 to 55.6% during the period of 1978 to 1979, then steadily rose to 58.1% during the period of 1986 to 1992 (Torrance et al., 2002).

A survey on obesity (BMI ≥ 30) conducted from 1985 to 1990 and through the period of 1994, 1996 to 1998 indicates a national prevalence of obesity that doubled from 1985 to 1998 (Katzmarzyk, 2002b).

In women, overweight and obesity was 33.9% from 1970 to 1972 and 42.3% from 1978 to 1979; however, from 1986 to 1992 it slightly reduced to 40.6% (Torrance et al., 2002).

- The number of obese individuals jumped from 5,300,000 in 2014 to 7,300.000 in 2018, which increase by 2,000,000 obese in three years. Besides, *the Epidemiology of adult obesity* stated that in 2016 the number of obese adult individuals reached 8.300.000, also it pointed out that the measurements of heights and weights (BMI) of adults indicated that obesity "increased more than 300% from 6.1% in 1985 to 26.4% in 2015/2016" (Obesitycanada.ca., 2020).

3.3. A.2.1   Trends in BMI

The following surveys relate to individuals aged 18 years old and above living in Canada who show a tremendous increase in BMI (Table 1). Along with the increase of obesity rate, the occurrence of obesity Class III rose from 0.4% to 1.3% from 1990 to 2003, which indicated an upsurge of 225% (Katzmarzyk & Mason, 2006).

- In 1998, the *CCHS* indicated that "50.7% to 61.2% of men and 39.9% of women exceeded the required plans for a healthy weight" (Tremblay et al., 2002). From 1994 to 1995 and 2000 to 2001, the *CCHS* indicated that there was a rise of 24% of obesity which went from "500.000 to nearly 2.8 million." This change meant that obesity reached 15% or approximately one person was obese in every seven individuals; this rise reached 13% from the six previous annual surveys (Statistics Canada, 2002).

- In 2000/01, the *CCHS* indicated that only 13 areas associated with *Montréal, Toronto and Vancouver* regions located in *Ontario, Quebec and British Columbia* had obesity levels lower than the NA of 15% (Statistics Canada, 2002).

- In 2004, 59% of individuals living in Canada were categorized as overweight or obese (Public Canada, 2018).

- In 2005, the *CCHS* indicated that the self-reported obesity rate was 15.9%, while the measured data was 24.2% (Public Canada, 2012).

- In 2007 and 2008, the *CCHS* indicated that the obesity rate was 17.4% according to the self-reported individuals (Public Canada, 2011).

- In 2008, the *CCHS* mentioned that the obesity rate was 17.2%, approximately 4.2 million were considered being obese (Statistics Canada, 2015i).

- In 2009, the *CCHS* indicated that 17.9% of individuals (self-reported) aged *18 and over*, approximately 4.4 million individuals, were categorized as obese. No modification of data occurred in the estimates from 2008 statistics. Nevertheless, statistics of obese men increased from 16% to 19% from 2003 to 2009, and obesity in women increased from 14.5% to 16.7% (Statistics Canada, 2015d).

- In 2010, the *CCHS* mentioned that 18.1% of individuals (self-reported) aged *18 and older*, approximately 4.5 million were categorized as obese. Quebec had 16.0% and British Columbia had 13.3%; both were a lower rate of obesity than the NA of 18.1%. Five provinces had a higher rate of obesity than the NA (Statistics Canada, 2015e).

- In 2011, the *CCHS* stated that 18.3% of individuals (self-reported), approximately 4.6 million individuals were categorized as obese. Quebec had 16.9% and British Columbia had 15.1%; both rates of obesity were lower than the NA, while seven provinces had rates of obesity elevated than the NA (Statistics Canada, 2013).

- In 2012, the *CCHS* mentioned that 18.4% of individuals, almost 4.7 million individuals, were categorized as obese. Two provinces had an obesity rate below the NA of 18.4%, specifically Quebec at 17.2% and British Columbia at 14.1%. Seven provinces had an obesity rate elevated than the NA (Statistics Canada, 2015f).

- In 2013, the *CCHS* indicated that 18.8% of individuals, almost 4.9 million individuals, were categorized as obese. Only two provinces had an obesity rate below the NA of 18.8% namely British Columbia at 15 % and Ontario at 17.9% (Statistics Canada, 2015g).

- In 2014, the *CCHS* indicated that 20.2% of individuals, almost 5.3 million individuals, were categorized as obese. Two provinces had a lower rate of obesity below the NA of 20.2% namely, Quebec at 18.2% and British Columbia at 16% (Statistics Canada, 2015h).

- In 2015, individuals aged 18 and over who self-reported to be obese were 26.4%, and 26.7% in 2016 (Statistics Canada, 2021b), but the *Epidemiology of adult obesity* gave 26.4% as obesity rate for the year 2015 and 2016 (Obesitycanada.ca., 2020).

- From 2016 to 2017, 27% of the individuals aged 18 and older living in Canada who (self-reported height and weight) were considered obese. Two provinces had an obesity rate lower than the NA, specifically Ontario at 26% and British Columbia at 22% (Statistics Canada, 2018b).

- In 2018, the *CCHS* indicated that 26.8% of individuals (self-reported height and weight), approximately 7.3 million individuals, were considered obese from the "reported height and weight that classified them as obese" (Statistics Canada, 2019e).

Moreover, other statistical surveys gave slightly different data namely:

- The Canadian Institute for Health Information (CIHI) indicated that in 2017and 2018 the obesity rate in Canada was 26.9% (Yourhealthsystem.cihi.ca., 1996-2020).
- The *statista.com.* (2021) indicated that the obesity rate in Canada was 26.1% in 2015; 26.5% in 2016; 26.9% in 2017; 26.8% in 2018; 27.7% in 2019 and 28.2% in 2020 (Www.statista.com., 2021).

Also, the overweight and obesity data from 2017 to 2018 are displayed in (Table A.3).

Figure 6: Contrasted Kids versus Adults Physical Inactivity, Sedentary Behaviors, and Fruits and Vegetable Consumption

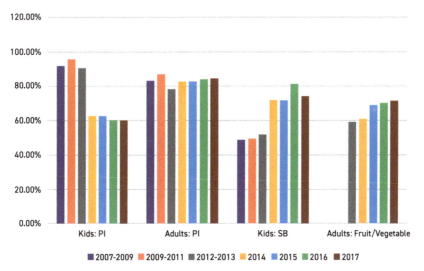

Kids: Physical Inactivity, Adults: Physical Inactivity, Kids: Sedentary Behaviors, Adults: Fruit/Vegetable Consumption

Source: Participaction.cdn.prismic.io. (2018); Public Canada (2017, 2019); Statistics Canada (2015ab, 2017ab, 2019a, 2020).

- In 2019, obesity prevalence continued to rise, 60% of individuals 18 years and above in Canada have been categorized as overweight or obese (Childhood Obesity Foundation, n.d.).

3.3. B   Key Health Risk Behaviors Contrasted with Medical Conditions

The data clearly shows (Figure 6) that overweight and obesity increased in conjunction with the increase of those *modifiable risk behaviors* (Public Canada, 2017).

First, the increase of physical inactivity as shown in the estimate does not take into account the age-standardized rate (ASR), which is the representative rate for two separated periods or geographic zones, the 2012 and 2013 *CHMS* indicated that beyond three quarters—approximately 77.8% or 20.1 million individuals in Canada aged 18 years and above failed to satisfy the Canadian *PAG* (Public Canada, 2017). Second, the sedentary behavior tends to be stable from 2007 to 2013, then it increased until 2018 (Participaction.cdn.prismic.io., 2018).

Table 2: Fruits and Vegetable Consumption Versus Obesity (2013-2017)

Years	National Average Rate for Fruit and Vegetable Consumption	Percentage of Obesity
2013	40.8%	18.8%
2014	39.5%	20.2%
2015	31.5%	26.4%
2016	30.0%	26.7%
2017	28.6%	27.0%

Source: Statistics Canada (2015abgh, 2017ab & 2018b, 2019a, 2021b).

Third, two surveys conducted eleven years apart confirm that individuals living in Canada have reduced their consumption of fruits and vegetables; the decline is around 13% according to recent research conducted by the University of British Columbia (Rolfsen, 2019) as shown in Table 2.

There is a significant decrease in fruit and vegetable consumption during the below consecutive years:

- In 2013 (40.8%)
- In 2014 (39.5%)

- In 2015 (31.5%)
- In 2016 (30.0%)
- In 2017 (28.6%)

  (Statistics Canada, 2015ab; 2017ab; 2019a).

Table 3: Healthy Behavior Scores by Province

Year & National Average	NB	NF	MB	YT	ON	QC	SK	AB	BC	NW	NT	NS	PEI
2015 - 50.9%	46.4%	36.6%	46.3%	-	49.4%	50.9%	45.1%	53.0%	57.3%	-	-	46.7%	50.9%
2016 - 51.5%	40.4%	37.2%	46.2%	51.5%	51.5%	51.5%	47.4%	51.5%	59.7%	51.5%	51.5%	46.4%	51.5%
2017 - 50.4%	43.4%	37.6%	50.4%	50.4%	50.4%	50.4%	46.0%	50.4%	56.1%	50.4%	50.4%	44.1%	50.4%

Source: New Brunswick (NB); Newfoundland (NF); Manitoba (MB); Yukon (YT); Ontario (ON); Quebec (QC); Saskatchewan (SK); Alberta (AB); British Columbia (BC); Northwest Territories (NW); Nunavut (NT); Nova Scotia (NS); Prince Edward Island (PEI) (Statistics Canada, 2017cd; 2018a).

3.3. C   Correlation of Health Rate Behavior with the Medical Condition of Obesity

Through HBS, the correlation of health behaviors and obesity can be evaluated (Table 4 and 5). Four parameters of behaviors are united into one score HBS; this correlation helps to determine the elevated degree of commitment to perform good *behaviors,* which is a requirement for every individual to carry their healthy lifestyle (Statistics Canada, 2018a). As previously mentioned in Chapter 3.3. A.1.4, HBS; there is an indication of only one or two provinces (Table 3) that show higher HBS than the national average score rate.

This fluctuation of HBS between higher and lower scores during consecutive years indicates a direct correlation of HBS with the increase of overweight and obesity (Statistics Canada, 2015abgh, 2017abcd & 2018ab, 2019ae, 2021b).

Figure 7: Healthy Behavior Scores by Province

Health Scores Behaviors by Province

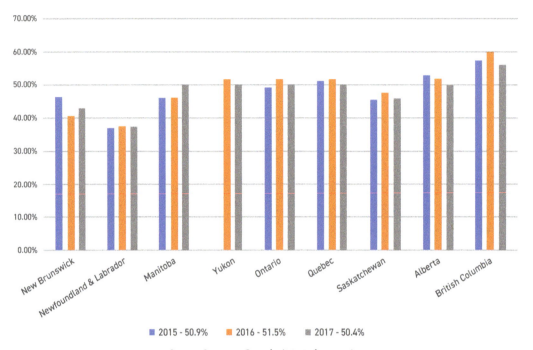

2015 - 50.9%   2016 - 51.5%   2017 - 50.4%

Source: Statistics Canada (2017cd; 2018a).

CHAPTER 4

RESULTS OF STATISTICAL ANALYSIS

4.1 Key Health Risk Behaviors Contrasted with Medical Conditions

Results from the statistical analysis shown in (Table 4) are described as follows:

1. Physical inactivity among children aged 5-17 who failed to satisfy the *PAG* during 2007-2009 (91.8%); 2009-2011 (95.5%); 2012-2013 (90.7%); as well as 49.8% of girls and 53.8% of boys who failed to satisfy the *PAG* (Public Canada, 2017). Due to the children's conditions of physical inactivity, the *Canadian Society for Exercise Physiology* (*CSEP*) has recommended parents to ameliorate the well-being and physical motions of babies and toddlers (Csep. ca., 2012).

   – During the 2014-2015 *CHMS*, 37.6% of children aged 5-11 and 12-17 years old met the *PAG* while 62.4% failed it (Public Canada, 2019).
   – During the 2016-2017 *CHMS*, nearly 60% failed the *PAG* versus 39.2% to 40% who met it (Statistics Canada, 2019b).

   The 2018 *Grade Benchmark* (*GBM*) for physical activity was D+ equal to or between 34% and 39% for children who met it, versus 60% of children who failed to meet the *GBM* (Participaction.cdn.prismic.io., 2018).

2. *Canadian Sedentary Behavior Guidelines* recommendation for children aged 5 years to 17 who failed to satisfy the requirement of the *SBG*:

   – 48.7% in 2007-2009; 49.6% in 2009-2011.
   – 51.8% in 2012-2013 (all genders).
   – 49.8% of girls and 53.8% of boys during 2012 and 2013 (Public Canada, 2017).

- 71.5% failed the *SBG* during 2014-2015 versus 28.5% who met it (Public Canada, 2019).
- In 2016, the *Benchmark* grade was F (19%) of children who met the *SBG* versus 81% who failed the *SBG* (Participaction.cdn.prismic.io., 2018).
- In 2017, the *SBG* percentage was not given; therefore, it could be calculated from the average between the 2016 *Benchmark* grade which was F (19%), and the 2018 *Benchmark* grade which was D (27% to 33%) giving altogether (F+D/2=19%+33%/2=26%); meaning that 26% met the *SBG* versus 74% who failed it in 2017 (Participaction.cdn.prismic.io., 2018).
- In 2018, only 35% of children aged 5 to 17 reached the expected *PAG* recommendation versus 65% who failed it (Participaction.cdn.prismic. io., 2018).

3. Adult physical inactivity of individuals aged 18 years old and above who failed to satisfy the *PAG*:
- The age-standardized rate (ASR) data for adults who failed to meet the *PAG* are as follows:
  - 82.9% during 2007-2009.
  - 86.6% during 2009-2011.
  - 78.2% during 2012-2013 (Public Canada, 2017).

The obesity rate was 18.4% in 2012 and 18.8% in 2013 (Statistics Canada, 2015fg).
- During 2014-2015, 82.5% failed the *PAG* versus 17.5% who met it (Public Canada, 2019).
- During 2016–2017, 83.6% failed the *PAG* versus 16.4% who satisfied it (Statistics Canada, 2019f).
- In 2017, 68.1% of individuals aged 18 to 34 made the only age group that highly accomplished the recommended *PAG*; 12 year-old children and above accomplished 57.4%; adults aged 35 to 49 accomplished 60.4%, and 50 to 64 adults reached 56.2% while individuals aged 65 and above reached only 40.6%, which was below the recommended *PAG* of 50% (Statistics Canada, 2020). Despite these self reported data of adults aged 18 and over, only 16.4% of adults as well as 39.2% of Children and youth met the *"physical activity target*

recommended in the Canadian 24-Hour Movement Guidelines during 2016-2017"; (Statistics Canada, 2019f).

– In 2018, 64.3% of individuals aged 18 to 34 accomplished the highest *PAG* requirement; 12 year-old children and above attained 54.6%; adults aged 35 to 49 accomplished 58.4%; and adults aged 50 to 64 reached 54.0%; while adults aged 65 years and above achieved only 37.3%, which was below the recommended *PAG* (Statistics Canada, 2020). Also, in 2018, 35% or approximately 40% of children aged 5 years to 17 reached the expected activity requirement (Statistics Canada, 2019f).

Table 4: Kids' Physical Inactivity versus Sedentary Behavior and Adults' Physical Inactivity versus Fruit and Vegetable Consumption

Year	Kids: Physical Inactivity	Adults: Physical Inactivity	Kids: Sedentary Behavior	Adults: Fruit/Vegetable consumption
2007-2009	91.8%	82.9%	48.7%	-
2009-2011	95.5%	86.6%	49.6%	-
2012-2013	90.7%	78.2%	51.8%	59.2%
2014	62.4%	82.5%	71.5%	60.5%
2015	62.4%	82.5%	71.5%	68.5%
2016	60.0%	83.6%	81%	70.0%
2017	60.0%	83.6%	74%	71.4%

Source: Participaction.cdn.prismic.io. (2018); Public Canada (2017, 2019); Statistics Canada (2015ab, 2017ab & 2019a, 2020).

4. Fruit and vegetable consumption surveys (Figure 8 and 9) conducted by the *CCHS* indicate that:
    – In 2013, 11.5 million individuals (40.8%) reached the expected recommendation of eating fruits and vegetables five times at least every day versus 59.2% who failed it.
    – In 2014, 11.2 million individuals (39.5%) met the recommendation versus 60.5% who failed it.

- In 2015, 9 million individuals (31.5%) met it versus 68.5% who failed it.
- In 2016, 8.6 million individuals (30.0%) met it versus 70% who failed it.
- In 2017, approximately 8.3 million individuals (28.6%) met it versus 71.4% who failed it. (Statistics Canada, 2015ab; 2017ab; 2019a).

Two surveys conducted by the University of British Columbia have discovered a fruit/vegetable consumption reduction of 13% (Rolfsen, 2019).

Figure 8: Fruits and Vegetable Consumption Versus Obesity (2013-2017)

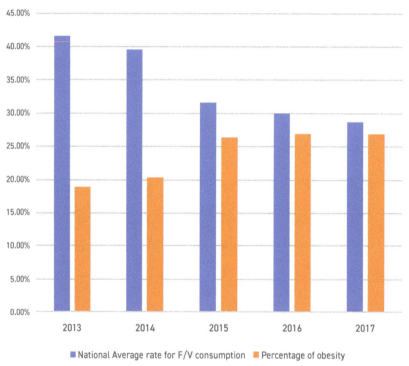

Source: Statistics Canada (2015 abgh, 2017ab & 2018b, 2019a, 2021b).

4.2   Correlation Analysis of Health Rate Behavior with the Medical Condition of Obesity

- In 2015, approximately 13.2 million individuals (50.9%) reached the expected HBS of 3 or 4. Only two provinces had an HBS above the NA of 50.9%. Six provinces had a lower rate than the NA (Statistics Canada, 2017c).

- In 2016, approximately 13.5 million individuals (51.5%) reached the expected HBS of 3 or 4. Only one province had the highest rate of 60% above the NA of 51.5% (Statistics Canada, 2017d).
- In 2017, approximately 13.4 million individuals (50.4%) reached the expected HBS of 3 or 4. Only one province had the highest rate of 50.4%, four provinces had a lower rate than the NA of 50.4 percent (Statistics Canada, 2018a).

Figure 9: Adults Versus Kids: Physical Inactivity and Sedentary Behavior; Adults: Unhealthy Eating and Obesity Rate

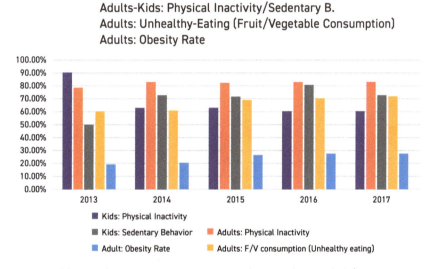

Source: Public Canada (2017, 2019); Statistics Canada (2015ab, 2017abcd & 2018a, 2019a).

4.3 Interpretation and Conclusion of Results

The results of the statistical analysis show the following:
- Very high physical inactivity among children and youth aged 5-17 years (Public Canada, 2017).
- Very high physical inactivity of adults aged 18 years and above (Public Canada, 2017).
- A considerable increase in sedentary behavior among children and youth in the last three years (Public Canada, 2017 & 2019).
- A significant decrease in fruit and vegetable consumption that confirms an increase in unhealthy eating in consecutive years (Statistics Canada, 2015ab; 2017ab; 2019a).

- Health behavior scores (Figure 7) show only one or two provinces that have an HBS above the NA rate in the last three years (Public Canada, 2017).
- The obesity rate has tremendously increased from 17.9% in 2009 to 26.8% in 2018 (Figure 4).

This increase of Health Behavior indicators correlates to the increase of obesity rate (Figure 7 and 8) as shown in the following data:

- 2009: 17.9%.
- 2010: 18.1%.
- 2011: 18.3%.
- 2012: 18.4%.
- 2013: 18.8%.
- 2014: 20.2%.
- 2015: 26.4%.
- 2016: 26.7%.
- 2017: 27.0%.
- 2018: 26.8%.

(Statistics Canada, 2013, 2015defgh & 2018b, 2021b).

Table 5: Two Health Risk Behaviors Contrasted with Obesity (2012 to 2013)

Health Risk Behaviors and Obesity			
Age of Canadians	Obesity (CHMS)	Unhealthy Eating (CCHS)	Physical Inactivity (CHMS)
12 to 19 years	12.6%	56.4%	90.7%
20 to 34 years	21.0%	61.0%	63.8%
35 to 49 years	29.2%	60.2%	82.0%
50 to 64 years	29.6%	63.6%	83.3%
65 years and above	26.0%	56.8%	88.2%

Source: Public Canada (2017).

CHAPTER 5

DISCUSSION

Several studies have confirmed that obesity is a behavioral disease (Katz, 2014; Sanders, 2017) that needs to be dealt with *health education* that targets the individual behaviors of each person or a group of individuals (Bandura, 2005; Jensen et al., 2013).

Globally, people live in environments where they get food easily but continue living a sedentary life, whereas some residential areas promote the local supply of healthy food and physical exercises, while other residences are high-risk obesogenic environments for their inhabitants (Elinder & Jansson, 2008).

Figure 10: Pathology of Obesity

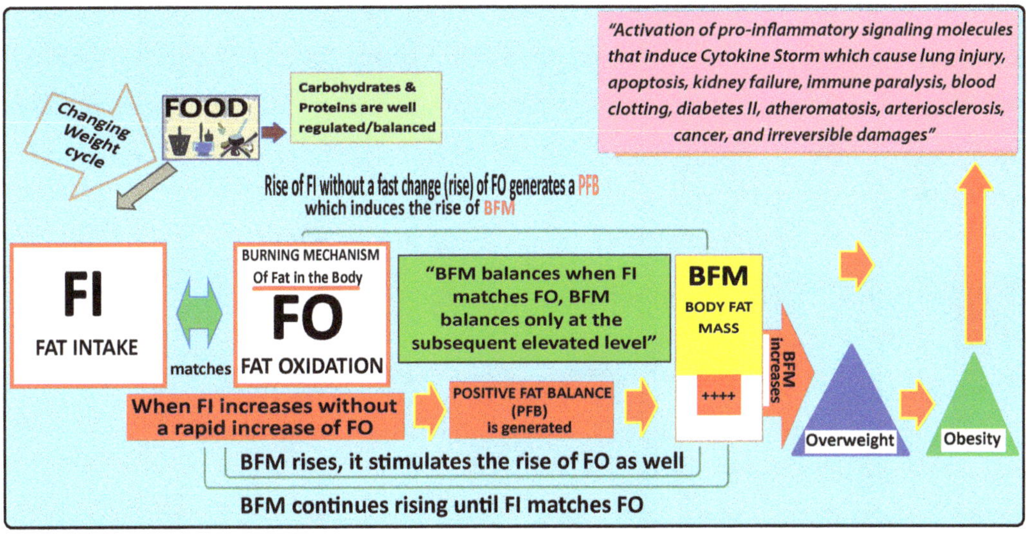

Source: Bing.com. (2007-2013); Bing.com. (n.d.a); Bing.com. (n.d.b); Bing.com. (n.d.c); Bing.com. (n.d.d); Flaquer et al. (2014); Johnson et al. (2012); Mandal (2019); Wensveen et al. (2015); Asghar & Sheikh (2017); Who.int. (2004); Zheng (2016).

Obesity is not completely acknowledged as a disease and it is generally described as a *lifestyle choice* (Halpern Bruno & Halpern Alfredo, 2014). Cases of obesity increased by 200% in all Canadian provinces from 1985; then, "21% of Canadians adults were estimated to become obese by 2019" (Twells et al., 2014). The reality is that in 2018 the obesity rate was 27% which reached 6% higher than the predicted rate 15 years earlier (Table 1) (Statistics Canada, 2019e).

The traced HBS have proven that unhealthy behaviors are elements of evidence that confirm the role of an individual as a causal agent of his medical condition of obesity (GlobeNewswire News Room, 2019; Obesitycanada.ca., 2019).

The results of statistical analysis show how weight of individuals continued rising, these facts indicate a continuous rise in obesity in all Canadian provinces, this rise of weight is the main problem that challenges public health in modern societies; this rise of weight could develop into a " grade 1 obesity which is not significantly associated with increased mortality, while the higher grades of obesity are significantly associated with increased mortality" (Flegal et al., 2013). The attention attributed to the social stigma concern stating that "fat is not the problem-fat, stigma is" (Bacon & Severson, 2019).

Nevertheless, fat is utilized as an eloquent sign to stigmatize other people, but it creates size discrimination and negative body image which should be resolved, and comfort should be given to those who are affected by this condition. Indeed, fat is already there; so, the thin will probably become fat in the future (Naafaonline. com., 1969).

The results of the statistics show a strong link of obesity to *individual behaviors*; particularly, "unhealthy eating and physical inactivity" (Who.int., 2004) and "sedentary behaviors" (Heinonen et al., 2013).

Those results displayed in Chapter 4 indicate the following:

1. Children aged 5 to 17, as well as adults aged 18 years and above, failed to meet the *PAG*.
2. Children aged 5 to 17 failed to satisfy the *SBG*.
3. A gradual reduction in fruit and vegetable consumption has been noticed and confirmed during consecutive years. This reduction has been about 13%.
4. The number of modifiable risk behaviors analyzed in Chapter 4 increased continuously in concomitance with the increase of obesity among adults (18

and above), concluding that obesity in Canada is linked to the *health behaviors* of individuals (Public Canada, 2017).

5. The HBS of 3 or 4 indicates that there were only one or two provinces that had an HBS above the NA score. Consequently, the overall fluctuations (NA versus provincial average) indicate a direct correlation of lower provincial scores with the increased body mass and obesity.

A link exists between neighborhood walkability and obesity (Colley et al., 2019), and it exists between "physical activity, lifestyle, and health" (Lukas et al., 1997). Genes do not work "in a vacuum" (Canada.ca., 2011). Metabolic factors alone could not be considered as major causes of obesity in Canada. These factors cannot work alone; they need other factors to empower them, particularly, the unhealthy risk behaviors of poor eating and not consuming fruits and vegetables, consuming food that contains an excess of fat, proteins, carbohydrates, on top of reduced physical exercises.

All these factors work together, or they have to be fueled by other risk behaviors such as sedentary behavior, heavy drinking, smoking cigarettes, and drug use.

Numerous studies have investigated the link between these activities and their impacts on the well-being of people. These studies have confirmed their link with the increase of sickness and mortality (Blaxter, 1990). Anderson (2004a) acknowledges that the change of our environment reflects the way people consume cheaper and available food, which is served in larger quantities, and frequently ingesting snacks that overload the body with excessive calories supplied in the daily diets.

Furthermore, junk food is freely obtainable in educational institutions at different convenient stores, which makes it difficult for children to choose healthy food (Blackburn-Evans, 2004).

Berall (2006) who treats obesity-related to Prader-Willi Syndrome realized that he could treat obese patients suffering from Prader Syndrome without any drugs by altering their diet and physical activity, which was enough to get a good result. He stated that even obese patients related to genetic causes respond to the alteration of diet and physical activity, and insisted that "once again, the environmental factors outweigh the genetics" (Blackburn-Evans, 2004).

He continued by saying that "if genetics were a significant factor, we wouldn't have seen this tremendous surge in obesity rates in the last generation. We have fundamentally the same genes we had 30 years ago; you don't get a genetic shift in that amount of time." He approves that one thing that changed is our environment. Nowadays, people live in a comfortable environment where food is offered anywhere, and the processing and delivery mechanisms are upgraded.

Some individual decisions and behaviors induce self-inflicted diseases which affect individual health, specifically "alcohol, smoking, sunbathing, eating a huge amount of fatty food" (123HelpMe.com., 2000-2018).

Even if behaviors are choices performed by individuals; indeed, they are manipulated by the "social, physical, and economic environments" of the working, learning, and daily living of the individuals (Public Canada, 2017). Obesity is an individual unhealthy lifestyle (Halpern Bruno & Halpern Alfredo, 2014; Katz, 2014) carried with excessive multiple HRBs (Public Canada, 2017) which involve the *self-inflicted character* of namely: choices, decisions, determination, motivation, stress, and impulsivity (GlobeNewswire News Room, 2019; Obesitycanada.ca., 2019) that promotes the *obesity epidemic.*

This self-inflicted factor (Jensen et al., 2013) negatively impacts strategies and intervention measures undertaken by the Ministry of Health in Canada (Sharma & Salas, 2018). Discussing how the same causal agent can apply self-initiated strategies to remedy their obesity will be the guiding key to uncover the role played by the individual behaviors in the "complex, chronic disease that has multiple contributing factors." Therefore, the cure will be to initiate individual "intensive lifestyle change" (Tello, 2017).

Since it has been established that obesity is the consequence of an *unhealthy lifestyle* (Lukas et al, 1997; Halpern Bruno & Halpern Alfredo, 2014; Sanders, 2017; Katz, 2014) carried with excessive multiple HRBs, which steadily induce the rise of overweight and obesity as confirmed by the statistical analysis in Chapter 4 (Public Canada, 2011; 2012; 2017; 2018; 2019).

This study has explored the link of an unhealthy lifestyle to overweight and obesity through:

1. The frequency of eating fruits and vegetables, which is required to supply
   anti-obesity nutrients to the body (Sharma et al., 2016), but the lack as well as
   the reduction of consuming them contribute to the development of obesity
   and other diseases such as heart disease and certain cancers (Statistics Canada,

2015ab & 2017ab). The reduction of eating fruits and vegetables are specifically emphasized in this dissertation as unhealthy eating; though, this term describes the lack of supplying required nutrients to the body such as sugar, fat, meats, vitamins, minerals, and enzymes, as well as overloading the body with the same nutrients. Unhealthy eating is emphasized in this paper because it involves fruit and vegetable consumption (one of the HRB) (Public Canada, 2017). By mathematical deduction, if 40% of people met the consumption target, 60% failed it.

2. The failure to satisfy the requirements of the *PAG* (Csep.ca., 2006).

3. The failure to satisfy the requirements of the *SBG* (The SBRN, 2011). This guideline indicates that children can be seated watching television, playing games, working on computers, or doing other leisure activities for two hours or less every day (Public Canada, 2019).

4. The failure to meet an HBS of 3 or 4, which was defined in the previous chapter to express what an individual should complete is as follows: "a person who smokes currently has (0); a person who is physically active for at least 150 minutes in the week has (1), not a heavy drinker (1), and eating fruits and vegetables five or more times per day (1), would have a score of 3 (0+1+1+1)" (Statistics Canada, 2017d).

Frontline doctors and obesity therapists can apply the cure that comprises behavioral methods of namely nourishment, physical exercise, and tackling emotional aspects that promote obesity (Tello, 2018). When targeting individual behavior (Halpern Bruno & Halpern Alfredo, 2014; Katz, 2014), it is required to apply health education.

This procedure focused on "a single individual or a group of individuals" (123HelpMe.com., 2000-2018), to treat obesity without any medical pill, but sufficiently dealing with the modification of the individual choices through the adoption of new healthy behaviors based on "Evidence-based guidelines" (Jensen et al., 2013).

Figure 11: Lifestyle Treatment Interventions

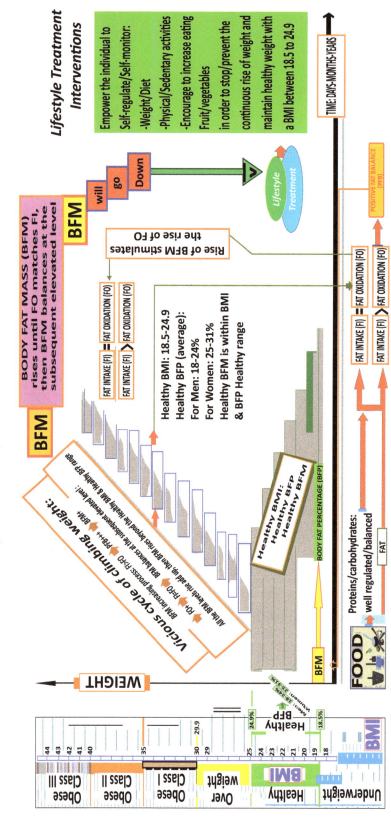

Source: Bandura (1997; 1998; 2005); Boeing et al. (2012) ; Colley et al. (2019); DiSalvo (2017); Halpern Bruno & Halpern Alfredo (2014); Kaplan (1992); Katz (2014); Jensen et al. (2013); Karin (2003); Kendra (2018); Lakerveld et al. (2015); Lev-Ran (2001); Maes & Karoly (2005); Mandal (2019); Mata et al. (2009); Patel & Hu (2008; 2012); Perron et al. (2012); Pugle (2024); Richard & Eduard (2000); Tello (2017); Vallerand (1997); Who.int. (2004).

CHAPTER 6

REMEDY OF OBESITY

6.1   Multiple Treatments for Obesity

Numerous applications have been utilized to treat obesity comprising of drugs, bariatric surgery, fighting fat by fat, behavioral treatment, and *lifestyle treatment interventions* as explained by MacLean et al. (2018). Brown fat has thermogenic properties that can have therapeutic roles, functioning through the "shifting of protons to a 'thermogenic pathway' rather than an energy-producing one which facilitates the uncoupling protein 1(UCP1), as expressed in the mitochondria of brown fat" (Lee, 2016).

6.1.1   Effects of Medical Treatments of Obesity

Still, trial and error is required to ascertain what medication has an effective effect on an individual. Most medications influence the functionality of the brain to process body mass control and how the brain cooperates with its surrounding. Nevertheless, the response to the action of the medication is individual; thus, some people react to the same medication differently. All types of treatments do not give the same result because some individuals' "weight loss surgery" can be an alternative (Tello, 2018).

Even if pharmacological agents have been found to have limitations, they remain useful weapons and are strongly stigmatized. To achieve long-term expectations, it has been established that there is a failure in administering short-term medications because of long-lasting and persistent disorders of obesity (Table A.1) which has been considered, nowadays, as a lifestyle choice and a challenge to be treated in the primary care setting. Furthermore, anti-obesity medications give fewer reduced weights than expected, and the misapplication of obesity medications for beautifying purposes, as well as the anti-obesity medications withdrawn earlier due to inopportune history

(Halpern Bruno & Halpern Alfredo, 2014). Seven million individuals in Canada are struggling with obesity; is it the lack of health resources?

The Canadian Obesity Network has cautioned that Canada missed delivering successful treatments of obesity (Chai & Tang, 2017). It was found that many anti-obesity drugs have unacceptable side effects, and many of them have been banned or disqualified because of undesirable side effects, as well as recent medications that have unknown harmful impacts on health. Some thermogenic medications that stimulate the sympathetic system, namely ephedrine and more others used as magic pills, are mostly related to elevated cardiovascular illness or linked to numerous psychiatric detrimental effects comprising of suicide (Halpern Bruno & Halpern Alfredo, 2014).

Unfortunately, procedures to stimulate energy outflow and produce heat in the body to deal with obesity have been found with total weight regain after a long period of the procedure. One has a detrimental health impact on the cardiovascular system (Kong et al., 2020); the second relates to *"the compliance with energy-restricted diet and consistent physical exercise"* to lower the *"metabolic drive"* that regains weight consequently to *"weight loss"* (MacLean et al., 2015). In common practice, if the individual is on a "maximal dose of the medication" and continues that therapy without any reduction of "5% of his initial weight during 12 weeks, the risk-to-benefit ratio" of that treatment is carefully checked and its discontinuation will be advised and implemented (Jensen et al., 2013). It is unfortunate that the "short-term use of anti-obesity drugs" will induce the regain of weight after discontinuation (Kang & Park, 2012).

6.2   Comparing the Medical to Non-Medical Treatment

It has been documented in the practical application of obesity treatments, specifically in a clinical setting and in the general literature, that "Clinical Perspectives on Obesity Treatment" have been found with dissatisfactions and shortage specifically in the current therapeutic procedures; various medical applications were ineffective to battle obesity, particularly the "pharmacotherapy, and bariatric surgery" (Heymsfield et al., 2018). Bandura (2005) said that colossal means have been spent in inopportune health customs, as well as overpriced pharmacotherapy. Anti-obesity medication failed to attain the expected results after therapy of long-term and repeated disorder of obesity (Halpern Bruno & Halpern Alfredo, 2014); as well, the deficit associated with the current implementation of therapy options for adults and children (Heymsfield at al., 2018); for that reason, a necessity to consider the *self-management model* is utmost because of the growing "shift from the medical management model centered on prescriptive regimens and compliance with them, to a collaborative self-management model" (Maes & Karoly, 2005).

This shift will tackle the *self-inflicted character* (Obesitycanada.ca., 2019) of obesity which has been described as an individual's *lifestyle choice* (Sanders, 2017; Katz, 2014). A *lifestyle choice* is an individual's "conscious decision to perform a behavior" (Study.com., 2003) that operates at the individual level. This individual-level influences or manipulates the obesogenic behaviors (physical inactivity, overeating, unhealthy eating, and sedentary behaviors) in obesogenic environments; subsequently inducing overweight and obesity (Lakerveld & Mackenbach, 2017). Unhealthy behaviors, specifically the obesogenic behaviors are consequences of individual choices (Katz, 2014 and Public Canada, 2017) which can sufficiently be addressed without any medical pill (Halpern Bruno & Halpern Alfredo, 2014) but with health education (123HelpMe.com., 2000-2018). The modification of the individual choices can be addressed with the adoption of new individual healthy behaviors based on evidence-based guidelines (Jensen et al., 2013).

6.3 Finding the Most Appropriate Obesity Treatment

Lifestyle treatment interventions will be considered as the "greatest self-management of health habits" (Bandura, 1998). The outset of these interventions indicates that lifestyle interventions are the first tools utilized by numerous clinicians to remedy and avert metabolic disorders linked to obesity, namely, "type 2 diabetes" (Osborne & Turner, 2019). These interventions ascend as an appropriate treatment model that involves the self-management that moves the therapy procedures from the "medical centered management" to a supportive "self-management model" (Maes & Karoly, 2005). Lifestyle interventions are "The Best Medicine You're Not Using" according to *Hippocrates* (460-377 BC) who stated the following: "If we could give every individual the right amount of nourishment and exercise, not too little and not too much, we would have found the safest way to health" (Karin, 2003). Lifestyle interventions will implement the strategic approaches leading to the adoption of change; then, change will educate the involved individuals to perform healthy behaviors that oppose over-weight and obesity (Jensen et al., 2013).

6.4 Can the Same Causal Agent Apply Self-Initiated Lifestyle Strategies to Remedy Obesity?

The individual becomes the causal agent of their obesity through the performed obeso-genic behaviors as detailed and proven by the results of the statistical analysis (Chapter 4). The Self-initiated lifestyle strategic approaches or intervention treatments are based on "social cognitive theory" (Bandura, 2005). Lifestyle interventions (Figure 11) aim to help the individual accomplish healthier *lifestyle choices*, to carry a healthy life in the future through "diet/physical exercises/sedentary behaviors" (Colley et al., 2019). These approaches can help any individual to specifically satisfy the demand to live a healthy life as an incentive mechanism that creates self-motivation (Bandura, 1998). Furthermore, the increase of self-control will help the individual to self-manage abun-dantly the vicious cycle (Figure 11) of their lifestyle customs to *"live longer, healthier, and slow the process of their biological aging system."* Then, a self-motivated individual will promote ways to manage their daily customs which are associated with their well-being (Bandura, 1997). Finally, through a progressive transformation induced by the socio-cognitive skills namely "self-control, self-regulation, and self-monitoring" (Bandura, 2005) which will empower the individual to overcome their unhealthy, challenging lifestyle. The individual will be successfully engaged in:

a. The adoption of goals guiding their efforts to combat obesity; indeed, with a clear judgment and prospect, they will redefine first, the goal to reduce over-weight and obesity (Jensen et al., 2013).

b. Second, they will initiate plans to increase self-motivation (Richard & Edward, 2000) to change their behavior (physical inactivity, sedentary behavior, drinking strong alcohol, and smoking) (Jensen et al., 2013).

c. Third, they will look for a way to modify or increase their self-reliance and hope.

d. Fourth, they will guarantee their "self-determination and freedom" (Richard & Edward, 2000) to execute a sequence of "self-regulation skills," namely the self-monitoring of their daily diet, which will have an increase in fruit/vegetable consumption and a very low-calorie content while they intensify physical exercises (Heymsfield at al., 2018).

How can these self-initiated strategies be implemented successfully to fight obesity? First, the individuals fix a specific goal to implement their lifestyle treatment; as they are empowered by all the pre-mentioned skills (Bandura, 2005); then, they can voluntarily initiate executing key tasks in an organized way as follows:

1. Self-regulate:
   - Nourishment: choosing well-adjusted healthy food according to their composition (oil, proteinic-sources, carbohydrates, alcohol, tobacco, drugs, and other medications) and control and limit the quantities and trace the discharges (feces, urines, and transpiration).
   - Increase fruit/ vegetable consumption (5 times a day).
   - Physical exercises: setting up timetables and plans for exercises, measure the intensity of training and its duration; then, control all physical motions (walk, running, working, standing, seating, and lying flat).
   - Sedentary behaviors: reduce or avoid car reliance, prevent technology dependency: internet, phone, computer-work that forces one to be seated.

2. Self-monitor: have monitoring forms to track:
   - Nutritional plan and track all physical exercises and movements.
   - Sleeping time: eight hours maximum to sleep in one day, avoid sleeping in a noisy environment, stay away from any source of disturbance (car noise, plane, animal barking, smoke, very hot or very cold environment).
   - Measuring daily weight (have a weight scale) to track change alongside physical exercise and feeding time.
   - Avoid sedentary behaviors: set a good schedule for children to control their screen time (watching television, gaming, or working on a computer), fix a time for leisure, promote walking, biking, and hiking.
   - Take drastic measures to manage the living environment (Figure 1), as re-designing the new healthy living environment that opposes the increase of weight: live with family members and friends that help reduce weight. Avoid heavy drinking (alcohol), reduce smoking tobacco if possible, avoid misuse of drugs that can affect the decision to apply *lifestyle treatment interventions* (Buddy, 2018). Avoid disturbing stressors that reduce total

sleep time or distressing conditions possibly comprising obesity (Patel & Hu, 2008; 2012; Perron et al., 2012).

– Identify and reduce the exposure to diverse obesogenic factors: domestic chemicals, food, medications (Table A.1), avoid exposure to smoke of cigarettes (Holtcamp, 2012).

– Have control over the accessibility to food (fast food, restaurants, high fat, and high calories drinks and snacks) (Elinder & Jansson, 2008).

Table 6: Overweight and Obesity, Men Versus Women from 2003 to 2013

Years	Overweight Men	Overweight Women	Obese Men	Obese Women
2003	41.30%	26.80%	16%	14.50%
2004	-	-	-	-
2005	41.20%	27.10%	16.90%	14.70%
2006	-	-	-	-
2007	40.90%	27.10%	17.90%	15.80%
2008	40.30%	27.40%	18.30%	16.20%
2009	40.20%	27.20%	19.00%	16.70%
2010	41.10%	27.20%	19.80%	16.50%
2011	40.20%	27.30%	19.80%	16.80%
2012	41.30%	26.90%	18.70%	18.00%
2013	41.88%	27.65%	20.09%	17.41%

Source: Statistics Canada (2015g).

CHAPTER 7

CONCLUSION

The conclusion can be drawn with the word of Tello (2017) stating that: obesity can be treated only with "Intensive lifestyle changes that involve knowledge and action," and Lakerveld et al. (2015) claim that the real therapy for obesity involves effective procedures that implement "self-control of physical activities and diet." However, overweight and obesity are consequently induced by "an energy imbalance between calories consumed and calories expended when used as energy by the body." Stable body mass can be sustained if the energy supplied into the body is identical to the energy burned. Once the supplied energy surpasses the quantity of burned energy, the exorbitant calories remaining in the body start stockpiling as fat, and sooner or later the body of the individual initiates accumulating weight leading to overweight and obesity (Mandal, 2019) as displayed in Table 6 & Figure 4.

Multiple HRB, such as physical inactivity, sedentary behaviors, unhealthy eating (huge consumption of sugar, fast food, meats, and reduced fruit/vegetable consumption) which promote the overweight and obesity as a consequence of an unhealthy lifestyle "Individual-level factors" (Figure 3). Always when someone wants to accomplish the true change, his motivation is required to direct all the processes of that change. There are many types of motivations, such as intrinsic motivation which is induced by *"Self-Determination"* (Kendra, 2018). Mata et al. (2009) stated that *"Motivational spill-over during weight control: increased self-determination and exercise intrinsic motivation predict eating self-regulation"*.

Then, Vallerand (1997) described such kind of motivation as a *contextual motivation* that has been related to a particular *life context* like physical exercises.

Consequently, *Lifestyle Interventions* have been considered effective because they are based on *"Self-Determination Theory"* which Richard & Edward (2000) describe in research that, this *"self-determination theory"* governs the surrounding circumstances in the community that enable *"versus"* prevent the normal practices of *"self-motivation"* and wellbeing of mental growth.

Self-determination enables individuals to preside over their *"choices, options, views and lives"* (Kendra, 2018). However, changing behavior requires a progressive transformation of individual customs which are entrenched in their mind, but their unhealthy behaviors are barriers (Bandura, 2005).

Strategic approaches called *lifestyle treatment interventions* (Figure 11) deal with such unhealthy lifestyles in terms of changing or reversing the role of each individual from promoting their overweight and obesity to the role of someone who identifies, understands, and modifies their environmental context (built, socio-economic, obesogenic factors) and implement regulation and monitoring of their diet and physical activities (Heymsfield at al., 2018). The *PAG* advises individuals aged 18 years to 64 to complete at least two hours and 30 minutes of reasonable to forceful intense "aerobic physical activity" every week (Csep.ca., 1967-2020).

Individuals have carried an *unhealthy lifestyle* for many years which became a great challenge to overcome in a *sustained long-term process,* such as modifying diet, exercise, habits, dependencies, or anything else (DiSalvo, 2017). The appropriate interventions will work only if the individual(s) come(s) to the point of setting reasonable goals, increase their "motivation (Richard & Edward, 2000), adapting their beliefs and hope," and tracking the implementation of a range of "self-regulation skills" particularly "self-monitoring" (Heymsfield at al., 2018). As the *self-inflicted character* of obesity is linked to the individual's unhealthy lifestyle; therefore, the effective endurance in these interventions will promote the scheduled transformation of behavior from an unhealthy lifestyle to a self-engineered therapy that will battle obesity (Bandura, 2005).

REFERENCES

1. 123HelpMe.com. (2000-2018). Self-Inflicted Diseases. [online]. Available at: www.123helpme.com/view.asp?id=114025 [Accessed 3 December 2019].

2. Abedi, M. (2018). Canadians aren't nearly as active as they think they are survey. [online]. Available at: https://globalnews.ca/news/4777241/canadians-physica-lactivity-survey/ [Accessed 19 March 2020].

3. Acasestudy.com. (n.d.). Descriptive Research Design: Definition, Methods, and Examples. [online]. Available at: https://acasestudy.com/descriptive-researchde-sign-definition-methods-and-examples/ [Accessed 24 December 2019].

4. Affenito et al. (2012). Behavioral Determinants of Obesity: Research Findings and Policy Implications, Journal of obesity, [PubMed] 2012: 150732. Available at: https://www.ncbi.nlm.nih.gov/pmc/articles/PMC3431098/ [Accessed 28 May 2020].

5. Anderson, H. (2004a). Program in Food Safety, Nutrition & Regulatory Affairs, U of T. [online]. Available at: https://www.childnutrition.utoronto.ca/faculty/harvey-anderson [Accessed 22 June 2020].

6. Anderson, H. (2004b). Harvey Anderson - University of Toronto. [online]. Available at: https://nutrisci.med.utoronto.ca/faculty/harvey-anderson [Accessed 8 April 2020].

7. Apovian et al. (2015). Pharmacological Management of Obesity: An Endocrine Society Clinical Practice Guideline. The Journal of Clinical Endocrinology & Metabolism, [online] Volume 100(2, 1), p. 342–36. Available at: https://aca-demic.oup.com/jcem/article/100/2/342/2813109 [Accessed 8 June 2020].

8. Apps.who.int. (2010). World Health Organization. Global recommendations on physical activity for health. Geneva. [online]. Available at: https://apps.who.int/iris/bitstream/handle/10665/44399/9789241599979_eng.pdf;jsessionid=9B39E3AD7668CE6A7AEBB8E2D9E801DC?sequence=1 [Accessed 23 May 2020].

9. Asghar, A & Sheikh, N. (2017). Role of immune cells in obesity-induced low-grade inflammation and insulin resistance. [online] Volume 315, p. 18-26. Available at: https://www.sciencedirect.com/science/article/abs/pii/S0008874917300345 [Accessed 21 June 2020].

10. Bacon, L & Severson, A. (2019). Fat Is Not the Problem—Fat Stigma Is. [online]. Available at: https://blogs.scientificamerican.com/observations/fat-isnot-the-problem-fat-stigma-is/ [Accessed 9 April 2020].

11. Ball, K & Crawford, D. (2006). Socioeconomic Factors in Obesity: A Case of Slim Chance in a Fat World? [online]. Available at: https://www.ncbi.nlm.nih.gov/pubmed/16928657 [Accessed 1 December 2019].

12. Bandura, A. (1997). Self-efficacy: The Exercise of Control. New York: W. H. Freeman and Company. [online]. Available at:https://www.worldcat.org/title/self-efficacy-the-exercise-of-control/oclc/36074515 [Accessed 30 March 2019].

13. Bandura, A. (1998). Health Promotion from the Perspective of Social Cognitive Theory. [online]. Available at: https://www.uky.edu/~eushe2/Bandura/Bandura1998PH.pdf [Accessed 30 March 2019].

14. Bandura, A. (2005). The Primacy of Self-Regulation in Health Promotion. [online]. Applied Psychology: An International Review, 2005,54(2), pp. 245–254. Available at: https://onlinelibrary.wiley.com/doi/abs/10.1111/j.1464-0597.2005.00208.x [Accessed 23 March 2019].

15. Banza, L. P. (2021a). (Banz5070@mylaurier.ca), 26 May 2021. Re: The family collection of pictures: Physical Exercises. Email to Cresap Research (kambok951@gmail.com).

16. Banza, L. P. (2021b). (Banz5070@mylaurier.ca), 26 May 2021. Re: The family collection of pictures: Eating Fruit/Vegetables. Email to Cresap Research (kambok951@gmail.com).

17. Banza, L. P. (2021c). (Banz5070@mylaurier.ca), 26 May 2021. Re: The family collection of pictures: Sedentary behavior. Email to Cresap Research (kambok951@gmail.com).

18. Banza, L. P. (2021d). (Banz5070@mylaurier.ca), 26 May 2021. Re: The family collection of pictures: Individuals drive Cars (lack of physical exercises). Email to Cresap Research (kambok951@gmail.com).

19. Banza, L. P. (2021e). (Banz5070@mylaurier.ca), 26 May 2021. Re: The family collection of pictures: Processed food. Email to Cresap Research (kambok951@gmail.com).

20. Ben-Menachem, Elinor. (2007). Weight issues for people with epilepsy—A review. [online]. Available at: https://onlinelibrary.wiley.com/doi/full/10.1111/j.1528-1167.2007.01402.x [Accessed 22 February 2024].

21. Berall, G.B. (2006). Prader-Willi syndrome | Canadian Paediatric Surveillance. [online]. Available at: https://www.cpsp.cps.ca/surveillance/study-etude/prader-willi-syndrome [Accessed 8 April 2020].

22. Bing.com. (2007-2013). Pathology of Obesity. [online]. Available at: https://www.bing.com/images/search?view=detailV2&ccid=5h3tNsE6&id=809023F0098A4A5625631E7687001C5084212527&thid=OIP.5h3tNsE6wp8W0roaCnsr-wHaFq&mediaurl=https%3A%2F%2Fi.pinimg.com%2Foriginals%2Ff5%2Fac%2F8c%2Ff5ac8ccbc2ea8529e39ecc43b73287f5.jpg&exph=584&expw=764&q=pathology+of+obesity&simid=608018393613271952&ck=E7C942E13CBED8C283C4621D6FF3D694&selectedindex=0&ajaxhist=0&vt=0&eim=1,6&sim=11 [Accessed 10 June 2020].

23. Bing.com. (n.d.a). Cytokine Storm – Bing. [online]. Available at: https://www.bing.com/images/search?view=detailV2&ccid=%2BP41ccKQ&id=23F-AF5583A87AC7459B383DE057CEF15C92D8A5A&thid=OIP.-P41ccKQ3AnfgwI17_Kk-wAAAA&mediaurl=http%3A%2F%2Fwww.sinobiologicalcdn.com%2Fstyles%2Fdefault%2Fimages%2FCytokines%2FCytokine-storm-cause.jpg&exph=566&expw=426&q=cytokine+storm&simid=608006878805428959&ck=8E30C5A08C707904736D8F35355403C2&selectedindex=2&ajaxhist=0&vt=0&eim=1,6&sim=11 [Accessed 21 June 2020].

24. Bing.com. (n.d.b). Cytokine Storm – Bing. [online]. Available at: https://www.bing.com/images/search?view=detailV2&ccid=3PSPc2TA&id=ABEB5499CD7149BF23B10B203D764F5290D8E44E&thid=OIP.3PSPc2TAWGapxxddsX9WIgHaFj&mediaurl=https%3a%2f%2fwww.sec.gov%2fArchives%2fedgar%2fdata%2f1175151%2f000114420412033733%2fimage_022.jpg&exph=525&expw=700&q=cytokine+storm&simid=607986834256298512&ck=DB0CA8A0DF41321676893C0AF57F15AA&selectedIndex=0&ajaxhist=0 [Accessed 21 June 2020].

25.   Bing.com. (n.d.c). Hyperplasia definition-Bing. [online]. Available at: https://www.bing.com/search?FORM=INCOH2&PC=IC06&PTAG=ICO-110497b3&q=hyperplasia+definition&uref=chmm [Accessed 7 June 2020].

26.   Bing.com. (n.d.d). Hypertrophy definition – Bing. [online]. Available at: https://www.bing.com/search?q=hypertrophy+definition&go=Search&qs=n&form=QBRE&sp=-1&pq=hypertrophy+definition&sc=8-22&sk=&cvid=9DE0208A48D54A14826CECCB79982C38 [Accessed 7 June 2020].

27.   Birch, L. L. (1999). Development of Food Preferences. Ann Rev Nutr. 1999, [PubMed] Volume 19, p.41–62. Available at: https://pubmed.ncbi.nlm.nih.gov/10448516/ [Accessed 4 February 2020].

28.   Blackburn-Evans, A. (2004). The Obesity Epidemic: Why are Canadians getting fatter? | EDGE Fall 2004. [Google Scholar]. Available at: http://scholar.google.com/scholar?hl=en&q=blackburn-evans+a.+the+obesity+epidemic:+why+are+canadians+getting+fatter?+edge:+how+research+works;+2004 [Accessed 5 April 2020].

29.   Blaxter, M. (1990). Health and Lifestyles. [online]. Available at: https://www.taylorfrancis.com/books/mono/10.4324/9780203393000/health-lifestylesmildred-blaxter [Accessed 9 December 2019].

30.   Block et al. (2009). Psychosocial stress and change in weight among US adults.Am J Epidemiol. 2009 Jul 15, [online]. Volume 170(2), 181-92. Available at:https://pubmed.ncbi.nlm.nih.gov/19465744/ [Accessed 27 June 2020].

31.   Bluher, M. (2009). Adipose Tissue Dysfunction in Obesity. [online] Volume 117(6), p. 241-50. Available at: https://www.ncbi.nlm.nih.gov/pubmed/19358089 [Accessed 14 April 2020].

32.   Boeing et al. (2012). Critical Review: Vegetables and Fruit in the Prevention of Chronic Diseases. [online]. Volume 51(6), p. 637–663. Available at:https://www.ncbi.nlm.nih.gov/pmc/articles/PMC3419346/ [Accessed 1 December 2019].

33.   Booth et al. (2005). Obesity and the Built Environment. I Am Diet Assoc. [online] Volume 105(5), p. 110–117. Available at: https://www.ncbi.nlm.nih.gov/pubmed/15867906 [Accessed 19 April 2020].

34. Borg, W. R & Gall, M. D. (1989). Difference between Descriptive and Experimental Research. [online]. Available at: https://pediaa.com/differencebe-tween-descriptive-and-experimental-research/ [Accessed 5 November 2019].

35. Bray, G. A. (2004). Medical Consequences of Obesity, The Journal of Clinical Endocrinology & Metabolism. [online] Volume 89 (6), p. 2583–2589. Available at: https://academic.oup.com/jcem/article/89/6/2583/2870290 [Accessed 22 November 2019].

36. Brewer et al. (1990). Social facilitation of the spontaneous meal size of humans occurs regardless of time, place, alcohol or snacks. [online] Volume 15(2), p.89-101. Available at: https://www.ncbi.nlm.nih.gov/pubmed/2268142 [Accessed 2 April 2020].

37. Buddy, T. (2018). How Heavy Alcohol Use Damages Memory Function. [online]. Available at: https://www.verywellmind.com/alcohol-damages-day-today-memory-function-62982 [Accessed 24 March 2019].

38. Burychka et al. (2021). Towards a Comprehensive Understanding of Body Image: Integrating Positive Body Image, Embodiment and Self-Compassion - PMC (nih.gov) [online]. Available at: https://www.ncbi.nlm.nih.gov/pmc/articles/PMC8323527/ [Accessed 24 February 2024].

39. Burton et al. (1985). Health Implications of Obesity: an NIH Consensus Development Conference. [online]. Available at: https://www.ncbi.nlm.nih.gov/pubmed/4031328 [Accessed 2 January 2020].

40. Byung-Cheol, L & Jongsoon, L. (2013). The roles of AT immune cells in the development of obesity-induced inflammation. [online]. Available at: https://www.ncbi.nlm.nih.gov/pmc/articles/PMC3800253/ [Accessed 23 June 2020].

41. Canada.ca. (2011). Obesity in Canada – Determinants and contributing factors. [online]. Available at: https://www.canada.ca/en/public-health/services/health-promotion/healthy-living/obesity-canada/factors.html [Accessed 12 September 2021].

42. Chai, C. (2015). Why your Car-Dependent Neighborhood is Increasing your Risk of Obesity. [online]. Available at: https://globalnews.ca/news/2109435/why-your-car-dependent-neighbourhood-is-increasing-your-risk-of-obesity/ [Accessed 5 May 2020].

43. Chai, C & Tang, V. (2017). Here's Why Canada gets a Failing Grade in Treating the Obesity Epidemic. [online]. Available at: https://globalnews.ca/news/3399779/canada-gets-a-failing-grade-in-treating-obesity-epidemic-report/ [Accessed 25 April 2020].

44. Cheng , V & Kashyap, S. R. (2010). Weight Considerations in Pharmacotherapy for Type 2 Diabetes: sulfonylureas, thiazolidinediones, and insulin are associated with weight gain. [online]. Available at: https://www.ncbi.nlm.nih.gov/pmc/articles/PMC2946585/ [Accessed 22 February 2024].

45. Childhood Obesity Foundation. (n.d.). Statistics - Childhood Obesity Foundation. [online]. Available at: https://childhoodobesityfoundation.ca/whatis-childhood-obesity/statistics/ [Accessed 2 April 2020].

46. Christakis, N. A & Fowler, J. H. (2007). The Spread of Obesity in Large Social Network Over 32 Years. N Engl J Med. [online] Volume 357(4), p. 370–379. Available at: https://www.ncbi.nlm.nih.gov/pubmed/17652652 [Accessed 19 April 2020].

47. Colley et al. (2019). An examination of the associations between walkable neighborhoods and obesity and self-rated health in Canadians. [online]. Available at: https://www150.statcan.gc.ca/n1/en/pub/82-003-x/2019009/article/00002-eng.pdf?st=zisx39x5 [Accessed 27 December 2019].

48. Croll, J. (2005). Body image and adolescents. [online] Available at: https://cmapspublic2.ihmc.us/rid=1JWW1ZDY3-11P9HDT-5HNV/body%20awareness.pdf [Accessed 28 May 2020].

49. Csep.ca. (2006). Canadian Physical Activity Guidelines - Background information.[online]. Available at:https://cdnsciencepub.com/doi/full/10.1139/H07-104 [Accessed 21 October 2022.]

50. Csep.ca. (1967-2020). Canadian Physical Activity Guidelines, Winnipeg. [online]. Available at: https://cdnsciencepub.com/doi/full/10.1139/apnm-2020-1109 [Accessed 21 October 2022.].

51. Csep.ca. (2012). Canadian Physical Activity Guidelines - Background information.[online]. Available at:https://cdnsciencepub.com/doi/full/10.1139/h2012-018 [Accessed 21 October 2022].

52. Darwish et al. (2020). The Influence of the Gut Microbiome on Obesity in Adults and the Role of Probiotics, Prebiotics, and Synbiotics for Weight Loss

- PMC (nih.gov). [online]. Available at: https://www.ncbi.nlm.nih.gov/pmc/articles/PMC7333005/ [Accessed 28 February 2024].

53. De Castro et al. (1990). Social facilitation of the spontaneous meal size of humans occurs regardless of time, place, alcohol or snacks. [online]. Available at: https://www.ncbi.nlm.nih.gov/pubmed/2268142 [Accessed 2 December 2019].

54. DelParigi. et al. (2006). Successful dieters have increased neural activity in cortical areas involved in the control of behavior. International Journal of Obesity, volume 31, p. 440–448. Available at: https://www.nature.com/articles/0803431 [Accessed 4 April 2020].

55. DiSalvo, D. (2017). 8 Reasons Why It's so Hard to Really Change Your Behavior. [online]. Available at: https://www.psychologytoday.com/ca/blog/neuronarrative/201707/8-reasons-why-its-so-hard-really-change-your-behavior [Accessed 17 March 2019].

56. Dyck et al. (2001). From "thrifty genotype" to "hefty fetal phenotype": the relationship between high birthweight and diabetes in Saskatchewan Registered Indians. [online] Volume 92(5), p.340-4. Available at: https://pubmed.ncbi.nlm.nih.gov/11702485/ [Accessed 15 September 2021].

57. Elinder, L. S & Jansson, M. (2008). Obesogenic environments – aspects on measurement and Indicators. [pdf] Volume 12 (3), p. 307–315. Available at: https://www.cambridge.org/core/journals/public-health-nutrition/article/obesogenic-environments-aspects-on-measurement-and-indicators/4D796A4002454DE633232704B3FE4219 [Accessed 25 November 2019].

58. Epstein et al. (2007). Food reinforcement, the dopamine D2 receptor genotype, and energy intake in obese and nonobese humans. Behav Neurosci. [online] Volume 121(5), p.877–886. Available at: https://www.ncbi.nlm.nih.gov/pubmed/17907820 [Accessed 18 April 2020].

59. Fawcett, k. A & Barroso, I. (2010). The genetics of obesity: FTO leads the way. [online]. Available at: https://www.ncbi.nlm.nih.gov/pmc/articles/PMC2906751/ [Accessed 18 November 2019].

60. Finkelstein et al. (2005). Economic causes and consequences of obesity. AnnuRev Public Health. [online] Volume 26, p. 239–257. Available at: https://www.ncbi.nlm.nih.gov/pubmed/15760288 [Accessed 19 April 2020].

61. Finne et al. (2013). Physical activity and screen-based media use: cross-sectional associations with health-related quality of life and the role of body satisfaction in a representative sample of German adolescents, [online] Volume (1), p. 15-30. Available at: https://www.tandfonline.com/doi/full/10.1080/2164 2850.2013.809313 [Accessed 28 May 2020].

62. Fitzgibbon et al. (2000). The relationship between body image discrepancy and body mass index across ethnic groups. Obes Res. [online] Volume 8(8), p. 582–589. Available at: https://www.ncbi.nlm.nih.gov/pubmed/11156434 [Accessed 19 April 2020].

63. Flaquer et al. (2014). Mitochondrial Genetic Variants Identified to Be Associated with BMI in Adults PLoS One. 2014. [online] Volume 9(8). Available at: https://www.ncbi.nlm.nih.gov/pmc/articles/PMC4143221/ [Accessed 9 April 2020].

64. Flegal.et al. (2013). Association of All-Cause Mortality With Overweight and Obesity Using Standard Body Mass Index Categories. A Systematic Review and Meta-analysis. [online]. Available at: https://www.ncbi.nlm.nih.gov/pmc/articles/PMC4855514/#:~:text=Relative%20to%20normal%20weight%2C%20both%20obesity%20%28all%20grades%29,overweight%20was%20associated%20with%20significantly%20lower%20all-cause%20mortality [Accessed 22 February 2024].

65. Frank, L. D. (2005-2021). President of Urban Design for Health. [online]. Available at: http://urbandesign4health.com/person/lawrence-d-frank [Accessed 12 September 2021].

66. Friedman, A. (2015). Architect and Professor School of Architecture, McGill University Montreal, PQ. [online]. Available at: https://www.mcgill.ca/architecture/avi-friedman [Accessed 5 April 2020].

67. Glass, T. A & McAtee, M. J (2006). Behavioral science at the crossroads in public health: Extending horizons, envisioning the future, Social Science & Medicine, Elsevier, vol. 62(7), p. 1650-1671. Available at: https://ideas.repec.org/a/eee/socmed/v62y2006i7p1650-1671.html [Accessed 6 December 2019].

68. GlobeNewswire News Room. (2019). Canadians with Obesity Treated as Second-Class Citizens Compared with Other Chronic Diseases: Report. [online]. Available at: https://www.globenewswire.com/

newsrelease/2019/04/23/1807669/0/en/Canadians-with-Obesity-Treated-as-Second-Class-Citizens-Compared-with-Other-Chronic-Diseases-Report.html [Accessed 5 November 2019].

69. Gordon-Larsen, P & Heymsfield, S. B. (2018). Obesity as a Disease, Not a Behavior. [online]. Available at: https://www.ahajournals.org/doi/10.1161/CIRCULATIONAHA.118.032780 [Accessed 28 November 2019].

70. GROSSMAN, B.(2010).Managing Adverse Effects of Hormonal Contraceptive associated with weight gain. [online]. Available at: https://www.aafp.org/pubs/afp/issues/2010/1215/p1499.html [Accessed 22 February 2024].

71. Gulati, P & Yeo, G. SH. (2013). The biology of FTO: from nucleic acid demethylase to amino acid sensor. [online] Volume 56(10), p. 2113-21. Available at: https://pubmed.ncbi.nlm.nih.gov/23896822/ [Accessed 17 April 2020].

72. Halpern Bruno & Halpern Alfredo. (2014). Why are anti-obesity drugs stigmatized? [online]. Pages: 185-189. Available at: https://www.tandfonline.com/doi/full/10.1517/14740338.2015.995088 [Accessed 3 October 2019].

73. Hammond, R. A. (2009). Complex Systems Modeling for Obesity Research. [online]. Available at: https://www.ncbi.nlm.nih.gov/pmc/articles/PMC2722404/ [Accessed 2 December 2019].

74. Healthypeople.gov. (2014). Nutrition, Physical Activity, and Obesity Across the Life Stages. [online]. Available at: https://www.healthypeople.gov/2020/leading-health-indicators/2020-lhi-topics/Nutrition-Physical-Activity-and-Obesity/determinants [Accessed 5 April 2020].

75. Heinonen et al. (2013). Sedentary behaviors and obesity in adults: the Cardiovascular Risk in Young Finns Study. [online]. Available at: https://bmjopen.bmj.com/content/bmjopen/3/6/e002901.full.pdf [Accessed 13 March 2020].

76. Heymsfield et al. (2018). Clinical Perspectives on Obesity Treatment: Challenges, Gaps, and Promising Opportunities. [online]. Available at: https://nam.edu/clinical-perspectives-on-obesity-treatment-challenges-gaps-andpromising-opportunities/ [Accessed 28 March 2019].

77. Heymsfield, S. B & Wadden T. A. (2017). Mechanisms, pathophysiology, and management of obesity. [pdf]. N Engl J Med. P, 376:254–266. Available

at: https://escholarship.org/content/qt63p9z787/qt63p9z787.pdf [Accessed 5 November 2019].

78. Hill et al. (2000). Genetic and Environmental Contributions to Obesity, Medical Clinics of North America. [online] Volume 84(2), p. 333-346. Available at: https://www.ncbi.nlm.nih.gov/pubmed/10793645 [Accessed 4 April 2020].

79. Holmes, D. (2022). High Altitude Health: Our cars are making us fat! [online]. Available at: https://www.eptrail.com/2022/03/19/high-altitude-health-our-cars-are-making-us-fat/ [Accessed 19 February 2024].

80. Holtcamp, W. (2012). Obesogens: An Environmental Link to Obesity. [online]. Available at: https://www.ncbi.nlm.nih.gov/pmc/articles/ PMC3279464/ [Accessed 28 March 2019].

81. Hrvatin, V. (2019). It costs Canada $9B to treat obesity, while barely any money is put into preventative care. [online]. Available at: https://vancouversun. com/health/it-costs-canada-9b-to-treat-obesity-when-barely-any-money-isput-into-preventative-care/wcm/ae78131c-7543-433b-aebb-14961916e803 [Accessed 27 November 2019].

82. Hruby, A & Hu, F.B. (2015). The Epidemiology of Obesity: A Big Picture. [online] Volume 33(7), p. 673–689. Available at: https://www.ncbi.nlm.nih. gov/pmc/articles/PMC4859313/ [Accessed 20 December 2020].

83. Huang et al. (2007). Body Image and Self-Esteem among Adolescents Undergoing an Intervention Targeting Dietary and Physical Activity Behaviors, Journal of Adolescent Health, [online] Volume 40(3), p. 245-251. Available at: https://www.sciencedirect.com/science/article/abs/pii/S1054139X06003843 [Accessed 28 May 2020].

84. Hu et al. (2003). Television Watching and Other Sedentary Behaviors in Relation to Risk of Obesity and Type 2 Diabetes Mellitus in Women, [online] Volume 289(14), p.1785-76. Available at: https://pubmed.ncbi.nlm.nih. gov/12684356/ [Accessed 28 May 2020].

85. Huvenne et al. (2016). Rare Genetic Forms of Obesity: Clinical Approach and Current Treatments in 2016. [online] 9(3), p.158-173. Available at: https:// www.ncbi.nlm.nih.gov/pmc/articles/PMC5644891/ [Accessed 17 April 2020].

86. Jensen et al. (2013). 2013 AHA/ACC/TOS Guideline for the Management of Overweight and Obesity in Adults: A Report of the American College of Cardiology/American Heart Association Task Force on Practice Guidelines and The Obesity Society. Circulation. [online] 129(25 Suppl 2): S102-138. Available at: https://www.ahajournals.org/doi/full/10.1161/01.cir.0000437739.71477.ee [Accessed 30 March 2019].

87. Johnson et al. (2012). The inflammation highway: Metabolism accelerates inflammatory traffic in obesity. Immunological Reviews. [online] Volume 249(1), p. 218–238. Available at: https://www.ncbi.nlm.nih.gov/pubmed/22889225 [Accessed 6 December 2019].

88. Kaplan, B. A. (1992). Health and Lifestyles. By Mildred Blaxter Pp. 268. (Tavistock/Routledge, London, 1990.) Paperback, [online] Volume 24(1), p. 139. Available at: https://www.cambridge.org/core/journals/journal-ofbiosocial-science/article/health-and-lifestyles-by-mildred-blaxter-pp-268-tavistock-routledge-london-1990-paperback/7C5C83540519EED7CDE3B7E2AB-F07A6D [Accessed 9 December 2019].

89. Kang, J. G & Park, C-Y. (2012). Anti-Obesity Drugs: A Review about Their Effects and Safety. [online] Volume 36(1), p. 13–25. Available at: https://www.ncbi.nlm.nih.gov/pmc/articles/PMC3283822/ [Accessed 9 April 2020].

90. Karin, B. M. (2003). International Journal of Epidemiology: Nutritional epidemiology—past, present, future. International Journal of Epidemiology, volume 32(4), p. 486–488. Available at: https://doi.org/10.1093/ije/dyg216 [Accessed 15 September 2021].

91. Katz, D. L. (2014). Perspective: Obesity is not a disease. [online]. Available at: https://www.ncbi.nlm.nih.gov/pubmed/24740128?dopt=Abstract [Accessed 3 December 2019].

92. Katzmarzyk, P. T. (2002a). The Canadian obesity epidemic: an historical perspective. Obes Res. 2002. [online] Volume 10, p. 666–674. Available at: https://sochob.cl/pdf/obesidad_adulto/The%20Canadian%20Obesity%20Epidemic%20An%20Historical%20Perspective.pdf [Accessed 22 May 2020].

93. Katzmarzyk, P. T. (2002b). The Canadian obesity epidemic, 1985–1998. CMAJ: Canadian Medical Association Journal, [online] Volume166(8),

p. 1039–1040. Available at: https://www.ncbi.nlm.nih.gov/pmc/articles/ PMC100878/ [Accessed 26 February 2020].

94. Katzmarzyk, P. T & Mason, C. (2006). Prevalence of Class I, II and III obesity in Canada. CMAJ: Canadian Medical Association Journal, [online] Volume 174(2), p.156–157. Available at: https://www.ncbi.nlm.nih.gov/pmc/ articles/PMC1329449/ [Accessed 26 February 2020].

95. Kazak et al. (2017). Genetic Depletion of Adipocyte: Creatine Metabolism Inhibits Diet-Induced Thermogenesis and Drives Obesity. [online]. Available at: https://www.ncbi.nlm.nih.gov/pubmed/28844881 [Accessed 5 June 2020].

96. Kendra, C. (2018). What Is Self-Determination Theory? [online]. Available at: https://www.verywellmind.com/what-is-self-determination-theory-2795387 [Accessed 30 March 2019].

97. Kong et al. (2020). Opportunities and challenges in the therapeutic activation of human energy expenditure and thermogenesis to manage obesity. [online] Volume 295(7), p. 1926–1942. Available at: https://www.ncbi.nlm.nih. gov/pmc/articles/PMC7029124/ [Accessed 26 June 2020].

98. Lakerveld et al. (2015). Successful behavior change in obesity interventions in adults: a systematic review of self-regulation mediators. [online]. Available at: https://www.ncbi.nlm.nih.gov/pmc/articles/PMC4408562/ [Accessed 17 March 2019].

99. Lakerveld, J & Mackenbach, J. (2017). The Upstream Determinants of Adult Obesity. [online]. Available at: https://europepmc.org/backend/ptpmcrender.fcg i?accid=PMC5644962&blobtype=pdf [Accessed 8 April 2020].

100. Laws et al. (2014). The impact of interventions to prevent obesity or improve obesity-related behaviors in children (0–5 years) from socioeconomically disadvantagedand/or indigenous families: a systematic review. [online]. Available at: https://www.ncbi.nlm.nih.gov/pmc/articles/PMC4137086 [Accessed 8 April 2020].

101. Lee, P. (2016). Wasting Energy to Treat Obesity. N Engl J Med, [online] Volume 375, p.2298-2300. Available at: https://www.nejm.org/doi/10.1056/ NEJMcibr1610015 [Accessed 8 April 2020].

102. Lev-Ran, A. (2001). Human Obesity: An Evolutionary Approach to Understanding Our Bulging Waistline, Diabetes/Metabolism Research Reviews.

[online] Volume 17, p. 347-362. Available at: https://www.ncbi.nlm.nih.gov/pubmed/11747140 [Accessed 5 April 2020].

103. Lindroos et al. (1997). Dietary intake in relation to restrained eating, disinhibition, and hunger in obese and nonobese Swedish women. [online] Volume 5(3), p. 175. Available at: https://pubmed.ncbi.nlm.nih.gov/9192390/ [Accessed 4 April 2020].

104. Lukas et al. (1997). The relationships between physical activity, lifestyle, and health. [online] Volume 33(2), p. 15-18. Available at: https://www.researchgate.net/publication/277324601_The_relationships_between_physical_activity_lifestyle_and_health, ICHPER Journal [Accessed 9 December 2019].

105. MacLean et al. (2015). The role for adipose tissue in weight regains after weight loss. Obes Rev 2015. [online] Volume 1, p.45-54. Available at: https://www.ncbi.nlm.nih.gov/pmc/articles/PMC4371661/ [Accessed 26 June 2020].

106. MacLean et al. (2018). Predict Obesity Treatment (ADOPT) Core Measures Project: Rationale and Approach. [online] Volume 26(S2). Available at : https://onlinelibrary.wiley.com/doi/10.1002/oby.22154 [Accessed 29 September 2021].

107. Madhubhashinee et al.(2017). Antipsychotic-associated weight gain: management strategies and impact on treatment adherence. [online]. Available at: https://www.dovepress.com/getfile.php?fileID=38063 [Accessed 22 February 2024].

108. Maes, S & Karoly, P. (2005). Self-regulation assessment and intervention in physical health and illness: A review. Applied Psychology: An International Review. [online] 54 (2), 245–277. Available at: https://asu.pure.elsevier.com/en/publications/self-regulation-assessment-and-intervention-in-physical-health-an[Accessed 22 March 2019].

109. Mandal, A. (2019). Causes of Obesity and Overweight. [online]. Available at: https://www.news-medical.net/health/Causes-of-Obesity-and-Overweight.aspx [Accessed 20 June 2020].

110. Mata et al. (2009). Motivational "spill-over" during weight control: increased self-determination and exercise intrinsic motivation predict eating self-regulation. Health Psychol. [online]. (28), pp:709–716. Available at: https://pubmed.ncbi.nlm.nih.gov/19916639/ [Accessed 16 March 2019].

111. Meijden et al. (2003). Determinants of Success of Inpatient Clinical Information Systems: A Literature Review. [online]. J Am Med Inform Assoc. p. 10(3): 23. Available at: https://www.ncbi.nlm.nih.gov/pmc/articles/PMC342046/#r13 [Accessed 5 November 2019].

112. Mobbs et al. (2007). Impulsivity is one of the factors responsible for obesity? [online]. Available at: https://www.ncbi.nlm.nih.gov/pubmed/17514924[Accessed 14 April 2020].

113. More, D. (2024). Can Antihistamines Like Allegra and Zyrtec Cause Weight Gain? [online].Available at: https://www.verywellhealth.com/do-antihistamines-cause-weight-gain-83094 [Accessed 18 March 2024].

114. Mosenkis, A & Townsend, R. R (2007). Antihypertensive Medications and Weight Gain-The Journal of Clinical Hypertension Volume 6, Issue 2 p. 90-90. [online]. Available at: https://onlinelibrary.wiley.com/doi/10.1111/j.1524-6175.2004.02847.x [Accessed 22 February 2024].

115. Naafaonline.com. (1969). We Come In All Sizes. [online]. Available at: https://www.google.com/search?q=Naafaonline.com.+%281969%29.+we+come+in+all+sized&tbm=isch&nfpr=1&hl=en&sa=X&ved=2ahUKEwixqpHM45rzAhXUqnIEHTEvCWkQvgV6BAgBEBE&biw=989&bih=459 [Accessed 9 April 2020].

116. Nam, S.Y. (2017). Obesity-Related Digestive Diseases and Their Pathophysiology. [online]. Available at: https://www.ncbi.nlm.nih.gov/pmc/articles/PMC5417774/ [Accessed 5 March 2024].

117. Nederkoorn et al. (2007). Impulsivity predicts treatment outcome in obese children. [online]. Available at: https://www.ncbi.nlm.nih.gov/pubmed/16828053 [Accessed 7 April 2020].

118. Neel, J. V. (1962). Diabetes Mellitus: A 'Thrifty' Genotype Rendered Detrimental by 'Progress'? American Journal of Human Genetics, [online] Volume 14, p. 353-362. Available at: https://www.ncbi.nlm.nih.gov/pmc/articles/PMC1932342/ [Accessed 5 April 2020].

119. Obesitycanada.ca. (2019). REPORT CARD ON ACCESS TO OBESITY TREATMENT FOR ADULTS IN CANADA 2019: Executive Summary. [pdf]. Available at: http://obesitycanada.ca/wp-content/uploads/2019/04/OC-Report-Card-2019-Eng-F-web.pdf [Accessed 5 November 2019].

120. Obesitycanada.ca. (2020). Epidemiology of Adult Obesity. [PDF]. Available at: http://obesitycanada.ca/wp-content/uploads/2020/08/2-Epidemiology-of-Adult-Obesity-4-FINAL.pdf [Accessed 23 March 2020].

121. Orlando, A. (2019). What's the Difference Between White Fat and Brown Fat? [online]. Available at: https://www.discovermagazine.com/health/whatsthe-difference-between-white-fat-and-brown-fat [Accessed 14 April 2020].

122. Osborne, B & Turner, N. (2019). Lifestyle Intervention - an overview | ScienceDirect Topics. [online]. Available at: https://www.sciencedirect.com/topics/medicine-and-dentistry/lifestyle-intervention [Accessed 10 April 2020].

123. Participaction.cdn.prismic.io. (2018). The 2018 ParticipACTION Report Card on Physical Activity for Children and Youth. [online]. Available at: https://participaction.cdn.prismic.io/participaction%2F38570bed-b325-4fc8-8855-f15c9aebac12_2018_participaction_report_card_-_full_report_0.pdf [Accessed 9 June 2020].

124. Patel, S. R & Hu, F. B. (2008). Short sleep duration and weight gain: a systematic review. Obesity. [online] Volume 16, p.643–653. Available at: https://www.ncbi.nlm.nih.gov/pubmed/18239586 [Accessed 8 April 2020].

125. Patel, S. R & Hu, F. B. (2012). Short Sleep Duration and Weight Gain: A Systematic Review. [online]. Available at: https://onlinelibrary.wiley.com/doi/full/10.1038/oby.2007.118 [Accessed 18 March 2019].

126. Penfold, S. (2004-2011). Penfold going to the hotdogs.[pdf].Available at: http://faculty.geog.utoronto.ca/Hess/Courses/JPG%201554%20Trans&UF/JPG1554%20readings/Week%203/penfold%20going%20to%20the%20hotdogs_Part1.pdf [Accessed 28 May 2020].

127. Perron et al. (2012). Review of the effect of aircraft noise on sleep disturbance in adults. [online] Volume 14 (57), P. 58-67. Available at: https://pubmed.ncbi.nlm.nih.gov/22517305/ [Accessed 17 March 2019].

128. Public Canada. (2011). Obesity in Canada – Determinants and contributing factors. [online]. Available at: https://www.canada.ca/en/public-health/services/health-promotion/healthyliving/obesity-canada/factors.html [Accessed 19 November 2019].

129. Public Canada. (2012). Obesity in Canada – Snapshot. [online]. Available at: https://www.canada.ca/en/public-health/services/reports-publications/obesitycanada-snapshot.html [Accessed 22 April 2020].

130. Public Canada. (2017). How Healthy are Canadians? - Canada.ca. [online]. Available at: https://www.canada.ca/en/public-health/services/publications/healthy-living/how-healthy-canadians.html [Accessed 3 November 2019].

131. Public Canada. (2018). Tackling Obesity in Canada: Obesity and Excess Weight Rates in Canadian Adults. [online]. Available at: https://www.canada.ca/en/public-health/services/publications/healthy-living/obesity-excess-weightrates-canadian-adults.html [Accessed 2 March 2020].

132. Public Canada. (2019). At-a-glance - The Physical Activity, Sedentary Behaviour, and Sleep (PASS) Indicator Framework. [online]. Available at: https://www.canada.ca/en/public-health/services/reports-publications/healthpromotion-chronic-disease-prevention-canada-research-policy-practice/vol-37-no-8-2017/at-a-glance-physical-activity-sedentary-behaviour-sleep-indicatorframework.html [Accessed 8 June 2020].

133. Pugle, M. (2024). HEALTH'S EDITORIAL GUIDELINES. [online]. AVAILABLE AT: BMI vs. Body Fat Percentage: Which Is a Better Indicator of Health? [online]. AVAILABLE AT: https://www.health.com/bmi-vs-body-fat-percentage-8424360 [Accessed 1 March 2024].

134. Rehman, A & Fry, A . (2023). Obesity and Sleep. [online]. Available at: https://www.sleepfoundation.org/physical-health/obesity-and-sleep [Accessed 5 March 2024].

135. Richard, M. R & Edward, L. D. (2000). Self-Determination Theory and the Facilitation of Intrinsic Motivation, Social Development, and Well-Being. [online]. Available at: https://selfdeterminationtheory.org/SDT/documents/2000_RyanDeci_SDT.pdf [Accessed 20 March 2019].

136. Roblin et al., (2017). Healthy Eating in Ontario: What Do we know about eating behaviors of Ontario? [online]. Available at: https://nutritionconnections. ca/wp-content/uploads/2021/03/Eating-in-Ontario-CCHS-2017-and-COVID-19_Mar_2021_Final-1-1.pdf [Accessed 25 June 2020].

137. Rolfsen, E. (2019). Canadians' consumption of fruit and vegetables drops 13 percent in 11 years. [online]. Available at: https://news.ubc.ca/2019/02/28/

canadians-consumption-of-fruit-and-vegetables-drops-13-per-cent-in-11-years/ [Accessed 30 April 2020].

138. Rosales, G. (2018). The true Causes of Obesity and society's ignorance. [online]. Available at: https://blog.obesityfree.com/the-true-causes-of-obesity-and-societys-ignorance [Accessed 5 April 2020].

139. Sanders, C. (2017). Manitoba Kids Tip Scales on BMI Trend: StatCan. [online]. Available at: https://www.winnipegfreepress.com/local/mani-tobakids-tip-scales-on-bmi-trend-statcan-438248013.html [Accessed 28 November 2019].

140. Seckl, J. R & Meaney, M. J. (2004). Glucocorticoid programming. [online] Volume 1032. P. 63-84. Available at: https://pubmed.ncbi.nlm.nih.gov/15677396/ [Accessed 4 April 2020].

141. Sharma et al. (2016). Paradoxical Effects of Fruit on Obesity. [PubMed] Volume 8(10), p.633. Available at: https://pubmed.ncbi.nlm.nih.gov/27754404/ [Accessed 22 June 2020].

142. Sharma, A. M & Salas, R. X. (2018). Obesity Prevention and Management Strategies in Canada: Shifting Paradigms and Putting People First. [online]. Available at: https://www.ncbi.nlm.nih.gov/pubmed/29667158 [Accessed 28 November 2019].

143. Sobal, J. (2001). Commentary: Globalization and the Epidemiology of Obesity. International Journal of Epidemiology, [online] Volume 30, 5 p. 1136.1137. Available at: https://academic.oup.com/ije/article/30/5/1136/724193 [Accessed 5 April 2020].

144. Statistics Canada. (2001). Annual Demographic Statistics. [Pdf]. Available at: https://www150.statcan.gc.ca/n1/en/pub/91-213-x/91-213-x2001000-eng.pdf?st=-54scaHe [Accessed 26 February 2020].

145. Statistics Canada. (2002). The Daily, Wednesday, May 8, 2002. Canadian Community Health Survey: A first look. [online]. Available at: https://www150.statcan.gc.ca/n1/daily-quotidien/020508/dq020508a-eng.htm [Accessed 26 February 2020].

146. Statistics Canada. (2013). Overweight and obese adults (self-reported), 2011. [online]. Available at: https://www150.statcan.gc.ca/n1/pub/82-625-x/2012001/article/11664-eng.htm [Accessed 22 April 2020].

147. Statistics Canada. (2015a). Fruit and vegetable consumption, 2013. [online]. Available at: https://www150.statcan.gc.ca/n1/pub/82-625-x/2014001/article/14018-eng.htm [Accessed 20 March 2020].

148. Statistics Canada. (2015b). Fruit and vegetable consumption, 2014. [online]. Available at: https://www150.statcan.gc.ca/n1/pub/82-625-x/2015001/article/14182-eng.htm [Accessed 20 March 2020].

149. Statistics Canada. (2015c). What's stressing the stressed? Main sources of stress among workers. [online]. Available at: https://www150.statcan.gc.ca/n1/pub/11-008-x/2011002/article/11562-eng.htm#a5 [Accessed 5 April 2020].

150. Statistics Canada. (2015d). Overweight and obese adults (self-reported), 2009. [online]. Available at: https://www150.statcan.gc.ca/n1/pub/82-625-x/2010002/article/11255-eng.htm [Accessed 23 March 2020].

151. Statistics Canada. (2015e). Overweight and obese adults (self-reported), 2010. [online]. Available at: https://www150.statcan.gc.ca/n1/pub/82-625-x/2011001/article/11464-eng.htm [Accessed 23 March 2020].

152. Statistics Canada. (2015f). Overweight and obese adults (self-reported), 2012. [online]. Available at: https://www150.statcan.gc.ca/n1/pub/82-625-x/2013001/article/11840-eng.htm [Accessed 23 March 2020].

153. Statistics Canada. (2015g). Overweight and obese adults (self-reported), 2013. [online]. Available at: https://www150.statcan.gc.ca/n1/pub/82-625-x/2014001/article/14021-eng.htm [Accessed 23 March 2020].

154. Statistics Canada. (2015h). Overweight and obese adults (self-reported), 2014. [online]. Available at: https://www150.statcan.gc.ca/n1/pub/82-625-x/2015001/article/14185-eng.htm [Accessed 23 March 2020].

155. Statistics Canada. (2015i). Adults who are overweight or obese in 2008. [online]. Available at: https://www150.statcan.gc.ca/n1/pub/82-625-x/2010001/article/11096-eng.htm [Accessed 27 February 2020].

156. Statistics Canada. (2017a). Fruit and vegetable consumption, 2015. [online]. Available at: https://www150.statcan.gc.ca/n1/pub/82-625-x/2017001/article/14764-eng.htm [Accessed 25 April 2020].

157. Statistics Canada. (2017b). Fruit and vegetable consumption, 2016. [online]. Available at: https://www150.statcan.gc.ca/n1/pub/82-625-x/2017001/article/54860-eng.pdf [Accessed 25 April 2020].

158. Statistics Canada. (2017c). Healthy behaviors, 2015. [online]. Available at: https://www150.statcan.gc.ca/n1/pub/82-625-x/2017001/article/14778-eng. htm [Accessed 30 April 2020].

159. Statistics Canada. (2017d). Healthy behaviors, 2016. [online]. Available at: https://www150.statcan.gc.ca/n1/pub/82-625-x/2017001/article/54865-eng. htm [Accessed 4 March 2020].

160. Statistics Canada. (2018a). Healthy Behaviours, 2017. [online]. Available at: https://www150.statcan.gc.ca/n1/pub/82-625-x/2018001/article/54975-eng. htm [Accessed 21 March 2020].

161. Statistics Canada. (2018b). Obesity in Canadian Adults, 2016 and 2017. [online]. Available at: https://www150.statcan.gc.ca/n1/pub/11-627-m/11-627-m2018033-eng.htm [Accessed 2 March 2020].

162. Statistics Canada. (2019a). Fruit and vegetable consumption, 2017. [online]. Available at: https://www150.statcan.gc.ca/n1/pub/82-625-x/2019001/article/00004-eng.htm [Accessed 21 March 2020].

163. Statistics Canada. (2019b). Physical activity and screen time among Canadian children and youth, 2016 and 2017. [online]. Available at: https://www150. statcan.gc.ca/n1/pub/82-625-x/2019001/article/00003-eng.htm [Accessed 5 March 2020].

164. Statistics Canada. (2019c). Canadian Health Measures Survey (CHMS). [online]. Available at: https://www.statcan.gc.ca/eng/survey/household/5071[Accessed 30 December 2019].

165. Statistics Canada. (2019d). Canadian Community Health Survey Data (2000 to 2011) Linked to the Discharge Abstract Database (1999/2000-2012/2013). [online]. Available at: https://www.statcan.gc.ca/eng/microdata/data-centres/data/cencchs-dad [Accessed 30 December 2019].

166. Statistics Canada. (2019e). Overweight and obese adults, 2018. [online]. Available at: https://www150.statcan.gc.ca/n1/en/pub/82-625-x/2019001/article/00005-eng.pdf?st=_vY8Q1ZY [Accessed 2 March 2020].

167. Statistics Canada. (2019f). Tracking physical activity levels of Canadians, 2016 and 2017. [online]. Available at: https://www150.statcan.gc.ca/n1/daily-quotidien/190417/dq190417g-eng.htm [Accessed 20 March 2020].

168. Statistics Canada. (2020). Physical activity, self-reported, adult, by age group, 2017 and 2018. [online]. Available at: https://www150.statcan.gc.ca/t1/tbl1/en/tv.action?pid=1310009613&pickMembers%5B0%5D=1.1&pickMembers%5B1%5D=3.1&cubeTimeFrame.startYear=2017&cubeTimeFrame.endYear=2018&referencePeriods=20170101%2C20180101 [Accessed 20 March 2021].

169. Statistics Canada . (2021a). Population estimates on July 1st, by age and sex, 2021. [online]. Available at: https://www150.statcan.gc.ca/t1/tbl1/en/tv.action?pid=1710000501&pickMembers%5B0%5D=1.1&pickMembers%5B1%5D=2.1&cubeTimeFrame.startYear=2009&cubeTimeFrame.endYear=2018&referencePeriods=20090101%2C20180101 [Accessed 12 September 2021].

170. Statistics Canada. (2021b). Body mass index, overweight or obese, self-reported, adult, age groups (18 years and older), 2015 and 2016. [online]. Available at: https://www150.statcan.gc.ca/t1/tbl1/en/tv.action?pid=1310009620&pickMembers%5B0%5D=1.1&pickMembers%5B1%5D=3.1&cubeTimeFrame.startYear=2015&cubeTimeFrame.endYear=2016&referencePeriods=20150101%2C20160101 [Accessed 15 September 2021].

171. Statistics Canada. (2021c). Body mass index, overweight or obese, self-reported, adult, age groups (18 years and older), 2017 and 2018. [online]. Available at: https://www150.statcan.gc.ca/t1/tbl1/en/tv.action?pid=1310009620&pickMembers%5B0%5D=1.1&pickMembers%5B1%5D=3.1&cubeTimeFrame.startYear=2017&cubeTimeFrame.endYear=2018&referencePeriods=20170101%2C20180101 [Accessed 17 September 2021].

172. Stigler et al. (2017). Mechanisms, Pathophysiology, and Management of Obesity. [pdf]. Available at: https://escholarship.org/uc/item/63p9z787[Accessed 20 November 2019].

173. Study.com. (2003). Lifestyle Choices and Personal Wellness: Decisions, Behavior & Prevention. [online]. Available at: https://study.com/academy/lesson/lifestyle-choices-and-personal-wellness-decisions-behavior-prevention.html [Accessed 9 April 2020].

174. Tello, M. (2017). Intensive lifestyle change: It works, and it's more than diet and exercise. [online]. Available at: https://www.health.harvard.edu/blog/intensive-lifestyle-change-it-works-and-its-more-than-diet-and-exercise-2017082112287 [Accessed 3 December 2019].

175. Tello, M. (2018). Obesity is complicated — and so is treating it. [online]. Available at: https://www.health.harvard.edu/blog/obesity-is-complicated-andso-is-treating-it-2018053013943 [Accessed 3 October 2019].

176. Tillotson, J. E. (2004). America's obesity: conflicting public policies, industrial economic development, and unintended human consequences. [online] Volume 24, p.617-43. Available at: https://www.ncbi.nlm.nih.gov/pubmed/15189134 [Accessed 2 April 2020].

177. The Sedentary Behaviour Research Network (SBRN). (2011). Canada Releases World's First Evidence-Based Sedentary Behaviour Guidelines | The Sedentary Behaviour Research Network (SBRN). [online]. Available at: https://www.sedentarybehaviour.org/2011/07/22/canada-releases-worlds-first-evidence-based-sedentary-behaviour-guidelines/ [Accessed 23 May 2020].

178. Tomalty, R & Mallach, A. (2009). America's Urban Future: Lessons from North of the Border. (Washington, DC: Island Press). [online]. Available at : https://islandpress.org/books/americas-urban-future [Accessed 15 September 2021].

179. Torrance et al. (2002). Trends in overweight and obesity among adults in Canada (1970-1992): evidence from national surveys using measured height and weight. [pdf]. Available at: https://www.nature.com/articles/0801991.pdf [Accessed 12 September 2021].

180. Tran. M. (2014). Obesity soars to 'alarming' levels in developing countries. [online]. Available at: https://www.theguardian.com/global-development/2014/jan/03/obesity-soars-alarming-levels-developing-countries [Accessed 4 November 2019].

181. Tremblay et al. (2002). Temporal trends in overweight and obesity in Canada, 1981-1996. [online] Volume 26(4), p.538-43. Available at: https://www.ncbi.nlm.nih.gov/pubmed/12075581 [Accessed 24 February 2020].

182. Twells et al. (2014). Current and predicted prevalence of obesity in Canada: a trend analysis. [online]. Available at: https://www.ncbi.nlm.nih.gov/pmc/articles/PMC3985909/ [Accessed 5 November 2019].

183. Twells et al. (2008-2021). Current and predicted prevalence of obesity in Canada: a trend analysis. [pdf]. Available at: https://www.researchgate.net/

figure/Predictions-of-future-prevalence-of-adult-obesity-in-Canada-from-2013-to-2019-by-weight_fig2_264389208 [Accessed 6 September 2021].

184. Vallerand. (1997). Toward A Hierarchical Model of Intrinsic and Extrinsic Motivation - LRCS. [online]. Available at: https://lrcs.uqam.ca/wp-content/uploads/2017/07/Vallerand1997.pdf [Accessed 28 March 2019].

185. Venniyoor. A. (2020). PTEN: A Thrifty Gene That Causes Disease in Times of Plenty? [online]. Available at: https://www.frontiersin.org/articles/10.3389/fnut.2020.00081/full [Accessed 12 September 2021].

186. Wensveen et al. (2015). The "Big Bang" in obese fat: Events initiating obesity-induced adipose tissue inflammation. [online] Volume 45, p. 2446–2456. Available at: https://onlinelibrary.wiley.com/doi/full/10.1002/eji.201545502 [Accessed 17 April 2020].

187. Wharton et al. (2018). Medications that cause weight gain and alternatives in Canada: a narrative review: Antipsychotics, antidepressants, antihyperglycemics, antihypertensives and corticosteroids all contain medications that were associated with significant weight gain. [online]. Available at: https://www.ncbi.nlm.nih.gov/pmc/articles/PMC6109660/ [Accessed 22 February 2024].

188. White, M. (2007). Food access and obesity. Obes. Rev. 8, [online] Volume 1, p. 99-107. Available at: https://www.ncbi.nlm.nih.gov/pubmed/17316311[Accessed 8 April 2020].

189. Whiteside, S. P & and Lynam, L. D. (2001). The Five-Factor Model and impulsivity: Using a structural model of personality to understand impulsivity. Personality and Individual Differences. [online] Volume 30(4), p. 669–89. Available at: https://www.sciencedirect.com/science/article/abs/pii/S0191886900000647?via%3Dihub [Accessed 23 June 2020].

190. Who.int. (2004). Obesity: preventing and managing the global epidemic: Report of a WHO Consultation (WHO Technical Report Series 894). [online]. Available at: https://books.google.ca/books?id=AvnqOsqv9doC&printsec=frontcover#v=onepage&q&f=false [Accessed 2 May 2020].

191. Who.int. (2021). World Health Organization. Obesity and overweight. Factsheet. Updated June 2016. [online]. Available at: https://www.who.int/news-room/fact-sheets/detail/obesity-and-overweight [Accessed 7 September 2021].

192. Wolf, A. M & Colditz, G. A. (1994). The Cost of Obesity. The US Perspective Pharmacoeconomics. [PubMed] Volume 5, p.34–37. Available at: https://scholar.google.com/scholar_lookup?journal=The+US+Perspective+Pharmacoeconomics&title=The+Cost+of+Obesity&author=AM+Wolf&author=GA+Golditz&volume=5&publication_year=1994&pages=34-37& [Accessed 22 March 2019].

193. Www.cbc.ca. (2015). Diabetes prevention is a job for architects, says professor Avi Friedman. [online]. Available at: https://www.cbc.ca/news/canada/british-columbia/diabetes-prevention-architect-architecture-1.3346364 [Accessed 12 September 2021].

194. Www.statista.com. (2021). Percentage of Canadian adults that are overweight or obese based on BMI from 2015 to 2020. [online]. Available at: https://www.statista.com/statistics/748339/share-of-canadians-overweight-or-obese-basedon-bmi/ [Accessed 15 September 2021].

195. Www.thefreedictionary.com. (2003-2020). stigmatization. [online]. Available at: https://www.thefreedictionary.com/stigmatisation#:~:text=stigmatisation%20synonyms%2C%20stigmatisation%20pronunciation%2C%20stigmatisation%20translation%2C%20English%20dictionary,disapproval%20-%20the%20act%20of%20disapproving%20or%20condemning [Accessed 24 May 2020].

196. Young, L. (2018). Canada's obesity rate has doubled since the 1970s. What happened? [online]. Available at: https://globalnews.ca/news/4456664/obesityin-canada/ [Accessed 8 April 2020].

197. Yourhealthsystem.cihi.ca. (1996-2020). 2017 to 2018: Adults (age 18 and older) considered obese based on self-reported height and weight (Percentage). [online]. Available at: https://yourhealthsystem.cihi.ca/hsp/inbrief#!/indicators/076/obesity-age-18-and-older/;mapC1;mapLevel2;/ [Accessed 23 March 2020].

198. Zheng et al. (2016). Mitochondrial epigenetic changes and progression from metabolically healthy obesity to metabolically unhealthy obesity: a cross-sectional study. Lancet Diabetes Endocrinol 2016, [online] Volume 4: Suppl 1: S16. Available at: https://www.thelancet.com/pdfs/journals/landia/PIIS2213-8587(16)30371-0.pdf [Accessed 9 April 2020]

APPENDIX A: TABLES

Table A.1: Drugs Promoting Overweight and Obesity

Some drugs are linked to weight gain such as:

Antipsychotics, antidepressants, antihyperglycemics, antihypertensives and corticosteroids

(Wharton et al., 2018)

Antipsychotic (Madhubhashinee et al., 2017)

Contraceptive drugs (GROSSMAN BARR, 2010)

Anti- epilepsy (Ben-Menachem, 2007)

Anti-diabetic (sulfonylureas, thiazolidinediones and insulin)

(Cheng & Kashyap, 2010)

Antihypertensive Medications (Mosenkis & Townsend, 2007)

Antihistamines (More, 2024)

Steroids drug (Data adapted from Apovian et al., 2015 by Heymfield et al., 2018)

Source: Ben-Menachem (2007); Cheng & Kashyap (2010); Data adapted from Apovian et al. (2015) by Heymfield et al. (2018); GROSSMAN (2010); Madhubhashinee et al. (2017); More (2024); Mosenkis & Townsend (2007); Wharton et al. (2018).

Table A.2: Physical Inactivity, Sedentary Behaviors, and Obesity

Year	Kids: Physical Inactivity	Adults: Physical Inactivity	Kids: Obesity	Adults: Obesity	Kids: Sedentary Behaviour
2007-2009	91.8%	82.9%	14.6%	24%	48.7%
2009-2011	95.5%	86.6%	11.8%	26.2%	49.6%
2012-2013	90.7%	78.2%	12.8%	26.5%	51.8%

Source: Public Canada (2017).

Table A.3: Overweight and Obese Individuals as Self-Reported by Age (18 years and above) during 2017 and 2018

Age group	Indicators	2017	2018
18 to 34 years	Overweight Obese	30.2% 19.7%	30.5% 18.7%
35 to 49 years	Overweight Obese	36.4% 28.9%	37.4% 30.3%
50 to 64 years	Overweight Obese	38.6% 31.9%	38.8% 31.3%
65 years and above	Overweight Obese	40.3% 28.0%	39.9% 28.1%

Source: Statistics Canada (2021c).

APPENDIX B: FIGURES

Figure B: Complications of Obesity

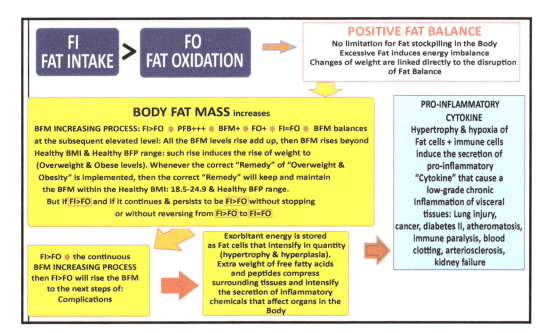

Source: *Asghar & Sheikh (2017); Bing.com. (2007-2013); Bing.com. (n.d.a); Bing.com. (n.d.b); Bing.com. (n.d.c); Bing.com. (n.d.d); Bray (2004); Byung-Cheol and Jongsoon (2013); Johnson et al. (2012); Lev-Ran (2001); Mandal (2019); Pugle (2024); Wensveen et al. (2015); Who.int. (2004).*

APPENDIX C: INTERACTIVE ACTIVITIES

Activity 1: Survey Questionnaires

These survey questionnaires aim to help the reader of the Book to *secure available and worthy resources that promote and schedule the transformation of the individual behavior* from *an unhealthy lifestyle to a self-engineered therapy* that battle Overweight and Obesity.

This Book brings awareness, individual lifestyle home-assignment and understanding about this *health concern called "Obesity". If really Obesity can affect everybody and risk ruining the entire life of the affected person, "Lifestyle Treatment Interventions"* has opposed it with the empowerment of the individual who should *self- regulate and self-monitor: weight/ diet, physical/ sedentary activities* in order to stop and prevent the continuous increase of weight.

1. What conditions are linked to the overweight and obesity condition?
    –   Weight increase: yes/no
    –   Unhealthy eating (reduced eating fruits/vegetables as well as overeating high calorie food): yes/no
    –   Increasing physical/sedentary inactivity: yes/no

2. How can overweight begin and develop into obesity?
    –   Everything begins with the interaction of *Obesogenic environment* and the o*besity-socioeconomic promoting factors*, which finally influence the *individual's lifestyle*: yes/no

3. How can this interaction overpower the *individual factors* (*Psychological/ Biological/ Genetics*)?
    –   The individual unhealthy choices determine the outcome: yes/no

4. Can a balanced lifestyle help to address the overweight's condition?
   – Yes
   – No

5. Why and how can any individual end-up performing *Obesogenic behaviors*?
   As long as the individual lives in a complex connection of both: obesity and socioeconomic factors that reciprocally stimulate each other or a common factor stimulates both. The individual carries an unhealthy lifestyle in an Obesogenic environment that intermingles with the Obesity-socioeconomic promoting factors (The different factors interact with each other at the same time): yes/no

6. Are young children also susceptible to develop overweight condition?
   – Yes
   – No

7. Are adults also susceptible to develop overweight?
   – Yes
   – No

8. Which one is the first activity that predisposes anyone to develop the overweight's condition? Yes/no
   – Diet: eating fruit/ vegetables; eating rich calorie food
   – Physical activities: running, deep breathing
   – Sedentary activities: seated watching television, playing games, working on computers, or doing other leisure activities for many hours.
   – Drinking hot alcohol
   – Smoking cigarette
   – Aging and becoming physically inactive

9. Should someone be physically active alone, with his wife, with his children or all the family?
   – Yes
   – No

10. Can someone be motivated to be physically active with the help of other people, such as his close family members?
    - Yes
    - No

11. Can someone need any help to balance his diet?
    - Yes
    - No

12. Can the diet be managed randomly or be scheduled and balanced according to its quality and quantity daily, weekly and monthly?
    - Yes
    - No

13. Can someone involve other family members to control his/ her diet?
    - Doing it alone: yes/no
    - Involve other people: yes/no

14. What can someone expect from other people as help to schedule?
    - The purchase of food (quality and quantity): nothing/ get advice
    - The type of meals-cooked and served: nothing/ get advice

15. How many meals can someone serve daily?
    - 1 time
    - 2 times
    - 3 or more times

16. How often can someone cook in his/her household daily?
    - 1 time
    - 2 times
    - 3 or more times

17. What type of food can someone buy and cook?
    - Vegetables
    - Meat
    - Grains

18. How many meals can someone serve daily?
    - 1 meal
    - 2 meals
    - 3 meals
    - 4 meals
    - 5 meals

19. How many liters of liquid (milk, juice, coffee, tea, water etc.) can someone drink daily?
    (1 cup = 1/4 Liter)
    - 4 to 7 cups
    - 8 to 11 cups
    - 12 to 15
    - 16+

20. In normal conditions, how many times can someone drink water?
    - 1 time
    - 2 times
    - 3+ times

21. How many meals can someone eat regularly everyday?
    - 1 meal
    - 2 meals
    - 3+ more meals

22. How much time can someone spend at the dinner table regularly?
    - Less than 50 minutes
    - Around 30 minutes
    - Over 1 hour and more

23. How many times can someone cook regularly food (per day/week)?
    - Per day:
        • 1 time
        • 2 times
        • 3+ times

- Per week:
  - 1 time
  - 2 times
  - 3+ times and more

24. Does someone need to be self-determined in addressing overweight and obesity concern?
    - Yes
    - No

25. What type of fast-food can someone order for his/her breakfast, lunch, dinner, snack/ dessert?
    - High Sugar
    - High protein
    - High cholesterol

26. Does Body Fat Mass (BFM) increase whenever a "Positive Fat Balance" is generated?
    - Yes
    - No

27. How many times can someone eat daily fruits and vegetables?
    - 1 time a day or
    - 2 and more (5) times a day
    - 7 times a week
    - 30 times a month

28. In Figure 11, the empowerment of the individual is achieved with the self-regulation and self-monitoring of weight/diet, physical/sedentary activities and the increase of fruit/vegetable consumption?
    - Yes
    - No

29. Is daily physical exercise good for someone to balance his/ her well being ?
    - Yes
    - No

30. How many times and how long can someone physically exercise (Walking/ running/yoga/ lifting weight)?
    – Daily:
    – Weekly:
    – Monthly:
        • 1 time: 10 minutes
        • 2 times: 20 minutes
        • 1: 30 minutes
        • 1 time: 1 hour

31. How much time can someone spend eating his/her favored meal on average?
    At the dinner table:
    – Less than 20 minutes
    – Around half an hour
    – Over an hour

32. How much pound of meat can someone eat in his/her daily meal?
    As a sedentary person: (0.1; 0.2; 0.5; 1; 1.5; 1.7) pounds:
    – More: yes/no
    – Less: yes/no
    – None: yes/no

33. How much tea-spoons of sugar can someone add to his/her daily beverage?
    – 1, 2, 3 or 4 tea spoon for breakfast
    – 1, 2, 3 or 4 tea spoon for lunch
    – 1, 2, 3 or 4 tea spoon for dinner
    – 1, 2, 3 or 4 tea spoon for dessert/ snack

34. How much dessert/ snack can someone eat?
    – 1, 2, 3, 4 a day
    – 1, 2, 3, 4 a week

35. How many hours can someone sleep regularly?
    – 6 or 4 hours a day
    – 8 hours a day
    – 10 hours a day

36. If someone wants to balance his/her own daily living, how many hours can he/she spend (watching TV, playing games, working on a computer, a phone: Being seated and using electronic devices)?
    – 30 minutes daily
    – 1 hour daily
    – 2 hours daily
    – 4 hours daily
    – 8 hours daily
    – 10 hours daily

37. If someone wants to balance his/her daily living, how long can he/she walk ?
    – 1 hour daily
    – 2 hour daily
    – 4 hours daily
    – 6 hours daily

38. Does it matter for someone to schedule or plan his/her physical activities that include all family members?
    – Yes
    – No

39. What conditions can disturb someone's sleeping time or habit?
    – Plane's noise: yes/no
    – Animal barking: yes/no
    – Smoke: yes/no
    – Drinking hot alcohol: yes/no
    – Drinking cold beverage: yes/no
    – Being exposed to a cold environment: yes/no
    – Being exposed to stressful conditions: yes/no

40. Is Fat oxidation the burning mechanism of Fat in the body?
    – Yes
    – No

41. Can someone reduce his sitting time by increasing his/ her physical exercises ?
    – Yes
    – No

42. Can someone increase his/her daily physical exercises in walking or riding a bike?
    – Yes
    – No

43. Is Positive Fat Balance generated whenever Fat Intake surpasses Fat Oxidation?
    – Yes
    – No

44. If someone dwells just 3 kilometers away from his/her workplace, does it matter for him/her to walk or bike to his/her workplace?
    – Yes
    – No

45. Does it matter for someone to consider reducing the consumption of high calorie-food (sugar-fat-meat)?
    – Rarely: yes/no
    – Sometimes: yes/no
    – Often: yes/no
    – Very Often: yes/no
    – Always: yes/no
    – Never: yes/no

46. Can someone consider these daily activities (eating fruits/ vegetables, physical exercises, sedentary activities) to be?
    – Critically important: yes/no
    – Somewhat important: yes/no
    – Slightly important: yes/no
    – Not important: yes/no

47. How long can someone perform these daily activities "laundry-work, kitchen chore, reading, playing games, computer work" in seated position?
    – How often:

- 1 hour: yes/no
- 2 hours: yes/no
- 6 hours: yes/no

48. What usual daily activities can someone perform in standing position (walking, working, leisure, reading, screen time)?
    - How often:
        - 1 hour: yes/no
        - 2 hours: yes/no
        - 6 hours: yes/no
        - 8 hours: yes/no
        - 10 hours: yes/no
        - 12 hours: yes/no

49. What activities can someone accomplish daily?
    - Working: yes/no
    - Rest at home: yes/no
    - Walking out door: yes/no
    - Drive a car/ ride a bike: yes/no
    - Shopping: yes/no
      How often:
        - 1 hour: yes/no
        - 2 hours: yes/no
        - 6 hours: yes/no
        - 8 hours: yes/no

50. What type of meals can a sedentary person make at home daily?
    - Fruits/ vegetables recipe: yes/no
    - Bread/ patisserie: yes/no
    - Meat/ Fish dishes: yes/no
    - High cholesterol dessert: yes/no

51. What home activities performed by someone who stays home daily? (working in the kitchen, cleaning the house, washing clothes, doing some mechanic repairs

(broken furniture) and displacing furniture/items in the house, working/walking in the backyard, walking in the nearby park or riding a bike):

– How often:
  - 1 hour: yes/no
  - 2 hours: yes/no
  - 6 hours: yes/no
  - 8 hours: yes/no
  - 10 hours: yes/no
  - 12 hours: yes/no

52. What physical activities such as:
  – Yoga
  – Running
  – Walking
  – Biking/ hiking

  can someone perform daily (At least during 150 minutes with deep breathing)?
  - Once daily or once weekly
  - Twice daily or twice weekly
    – How often:
      - 1 hour: yes/no
      - 2 hours: yes/no
      - 6 hours: yes/no
      - 8 hours: yes/no
      - 10 hours: yes/no
      - 12 hours: yes/no

53. Usually, who initiates physical activities in most families?
  – Father: yes/no
  – Mother: yes/no
  – Children: yes/no

54. Does it matter for anyone to regularly measure his/her weight: daily, weekly or monthly?
  – Yes
  – No

55. In Mr. John's life (Book, page 21), there are facts showing that he is very busy: yes/no

He is free to carry his unhealthy lifestyle: yes/no

A: If "free-unhealthy-choices-insecure life" are represented by a left-side glove or hand; therefore, "free-healthy-choices-secure life" will be displayed by a right-side glove or hand outstretched in all circumstances to greet. Nobody shakes hand with a left hand (left-side glove); always shaking hand is completed with overstretched right hand to greet.

   – Are free-healthy-choices the responsibility of each individual? Yes/no
   – Are the family members, also responsible to help carrying healthy life? Yes/no
   – Do healthy choices concern everybody?
   – Yes
   – No

56. Is daily life affected by different obesogenic factors such as: the *"Obesogenic Environment"*, *"Obesity socioeconomic promoting factors* and *Obesogenic lifestyle behaviors"*?

   – Yes
   – No

That can promote overweight and obesity?

   – Yes
   – No

A: How can these factors (Obesogenic Environment) promote someone's overweight and obesity?

   – Indoor: yes/no
   – Outdoor: yes/no

Can someone create an *Obesogenic Environment*?

   – Yes
   – No

B: Can the *"Obesity-socioeconomic promoting factors"* be associated with someone's living activity?

   – Indoor: yes/no
   – Outdoor: yes/no

Who are affected by these "obesity-socioeconomic promoting factors"?

– Everybody: yes/no

– Parents: yes/no

– Children: yes/no

C: What are lifestyle behaviors that can be linked to overweight and obesity?

– Unhealthy eating and

– Physical inactivity/sedentary behavior: (screen time devices/ technology: watching TV, playing games, working on a computer, a phone while being seated): yes/no

D: Can some dietary behaviors and some *Obesogenic Environment* promote conjunctly overweight and obesity?

– Yes

– No

E: Can some occupational status, education and income promote the happening of overweight/ obesity?

– Yes

– No

F: Who can be affected by these lifestyle behaviors?

– Father: yes/no

– Mother: yes/no

– Children: yes/no

– All the family members: yes/no

57. Can everybody consider *"Lifestyle treatment interventions"* as the "greatest self-management of health habits"?

– Yes

– No

58. Can everybody consider the "self-management model of overweight" to be much supportive and effective in the long journey to reduce overweight?

– Yes

– No

59. Long-time ago: *Hippocrates* (460-377 BC) stated the following: "If we could give every individual the right amount of nourishment and exercise, not too little and not too much" will be "The Best Medicine You're Not Using."

Does anyone agree that " the Hippocrates' statement teaches and remains always the safest way to health?"
   - Yes
   - No

60. If really *"Lifestyle treatment interventions"* empower the individual to *conclusively* change his *life habits in order to bring down his weight/obesity* through regulation and monitoring of their diet/ physical and sedentary activities and boosting the consumption of fruit/vegetables:
   - Yes
   - No

61. Is it true that *Lifestyle interventions* aim to help the individual accomplishing healthier *lifestyle choices*, to carry a healthy life in the future?
   - Yes
   - No

62. Does Figure 11 need to be positioned correctly in order to read it easily? Yes/No
   - If yes, the same way anyone will need to correctly fix his/her "environment, socio-economic customs and living style choices" to live a healthy lifestyle.

63. After answering to all the questions above: Can anyone take drastic action to stop and prevent the increase of weight?
   - Can surely everybody be involved in the fight against the overweight and obesity?
      - Yes
      - No

Activity 2: Word search Puzzle-Games

RULES FOR PLAYING THE GAMES

HIDDEN WORDS IN THE BOXES CAN BE FOUND IN MANY DIRECTIONS:
- – HORIZONTALLY: FORWARD AND BACKWARD
- – VERTICALLY: DOWN, UP
- – LEFTSLANTING: UP & DOWN
- – RIGHTSLANTING: UP & DOWN

SOME WORDS CAN BE ENCIRCLED FOLLOWING THE
ABOVE DIRECTIONS

Word search Puzzle-Game A

M	W	A	E	C	N	E	D	N	E	P	E	D	R	A	C	D	T	L
A	I	T	G	N	I	D	N	U	O	R	R	U	S	I	V	E	S	I
N	T	N	Y	R	A	T	N	E	D	E	S	N	M	K	G	A	M	V
Y	H	E	D	E	S	A	E	R	C	N	I	O	E	V	I	L	S	I
F	E	M	T	S	E	C	I	V	E	D	N	T	W	O	R	K	I	N
A	G	P	R	E	D	U	C	E	D	O	N	A	H	G	I	H	N	G
C	N	O	P	E	O	P	L	E	A	D	L	L	I	T	S	A	C	
T	A	L	K	K	C	A	L	E	C	K	S	T	O	R	E	S	H	I
O	H	E	H	C	I	H	W	A	A	A	C	C	E	S	S	M	C	M
R	C	V	T	H	A	T	M	B	I	G	Y	L	P	P	U	S	E	O
S	E	E	A	O	O	E	I	D	O	O	F	B	K	S	I	R	M	N
I	H	D	R	A	E	L	E	C	T	R	O	N	I	C	D	O	G	O
N	T	N	E	V	I	T	Y	T	I	L	I	B	A	P	A	C	N	C
C	F	A	E	T	W	I	D	E	R	E	A	C	H	I	N	G	I	E
L	R	D	Y	Y	L	T	N	E	U	Q	E	S	B	U	S	C	S	A
U	E	N	O	I	T	P	M	U	S	N	O	C	R	E	V	O	S	S
D	E	L	A	C	I	S	Y	H	P	E	I	R	O	L	A	C	E	I
E	N	O	T	C	I	N	E	G	O	S	E	B	O	L	O	O	C	N
E	N	V	I	R	O	N	M	E	N	T	S	S	E	N	E	G	O	A
D	E	D	A	R	G	P	U	S	Y	T	I	V	I	T	C	A	R	O
D	E	L	I	V	E	R	Y	V	A	C	U	U	M	I	S	S	P	S

ENCIRCLE ANY WORD IN THE ABOVE PUZZLE WHICH IS SIMILAR TO ANY BELOW WORD:

1. THE CHANGE OF THE ENVIRONMENT WHICH CAME WITH THE ECONOMIC DEVELOPMENT THAT REDUCED WALKABILITY AND INCREASED SEDENTARY ACTIVITY, AND SUBSEQUENTLY INCREASED A WIDE-REACHING CAPABILITY OF FOOD SUPPLY WHICH INCREASED ACCESS TO THE SURROUNDING STORES OF FOOD AND THE "OVER-CONSUMPTION" OF HIGH CALORIE FOOD AND A LACK OF PHYSICAL ACTIVITY. AS PEOPLE STILL LIVE IN "HIGH-RISK OBESOGENIC ENVIRONMENTS WITH ELECTRONIC DEVICES AND CAR-DEPENDENCE", AND MANY OBESOGENIC FACTORS THAT INCLUDE THE UPGRADED PROCESSING AND DELIVERY MECHANISMS OF FOOD; SO, GENES DO NOT WORK "IN A VACUUM"
2. EXTRA WORDS: GET, FREE, LEAD, NOT, MISS, COOL, BIG, DEAL

OBESITY

Word search Puzzle-Game B

E	V	E	R	Y	L	A	U	D	I	V	I	D	N	I	N	A
Y	L	T	N	E	D	I	V	E	Y	H	T	L	A	E	H	D
C	S	E	N	I	L	E	D	I	U	G	S	R	T	I	E	U
A	N	Y	T	I	V	I	T	C	A	T	O	U	S	E	R	L
N	L	A	C	I	S	Y	H	P	N	E	H	T	H	A	T	T
E	D	E	P	O	L	E	V	E	D	F	O	U	R	U	N	S
W	T	E	E	R	H	T	M	L	I	F	E	S	T	Y	L	E
R	O	I	V	A	H	E	B	S	E	D	E	N	T	A	R	Y
S	E	G	A	P	R	O	G	R	E	S	S	I	V	E	L	Y
R	O	T	N	I	O	L	S	A	T	I	S	F	Y	N	A	C
D	N	A	U	N	F	A	I	L	U	R	E	S	E	H	T	O
N	A	Q	N	A	G	E	B	V	L	L	A	E	M	I	T	N
S	E	M	E	E	T	E	C	H	I	L	D	R	E	N	A	F
R	S	W	I	F	T	L	Y	W	E	N	S	C	O	R	E	I
F	O	T	F	O	R	S	O	M	E	B	G	F	O	O	D	R
G	E	N	E	R	A	T	I	O	N	S	L	L	I	W	E	M
O	T	N	E	G	A	Y	L	L	A	I	T	N	E	T	O	P
Y	T	I	S	E	B	O	L	A	S	U	A	C	A	N	W	O
E	R	U	T	U	F	E	L	A	C	S	T	N	I	O	P	N

ENCIRCLE ANY WORD IN THE ABOVE PUZZLE WHICH IS SIMILAR TO ANY BELOW WORD:
1. THE FAILURE TO SATISFY SOME HEALTHY LIVING REQUIREMENTS:
2. SWIFTLY BEGAN AND PROGRESSIVELY DEVELOPED INTO A NEW LIFESTYLE FOR FUTURE GENERATIONS OF ALL AGES:
3. FOR CHILDREN: FAILURE TO SATISFY THE REQUIREMENTS OF THE PHYSICAL ACTIVITY GUIDELINES, AND SEDENTARY BEHAVIOR GUIDELINES
4. FOR ADULTS: FAILURE TO MEET AN HEALTHY BEHAVIOR SCORE OF THREE OR FOUR-POINT ON THE SCALE, ALL THESE FAILURES WILL CONFIRM EVIDENTLY THAT EVERY INDIVIDUAL CAN POTENTIALLY BE THE CAUSAL AGENT OF HIS OR HER OWN OBESITY
5. EXTRA WORDS: IN, TIME, WE, EAT, FOOD, THEN, GO, TO, RUN

Word search Puzzle-Game C

S	R	S	I	K	C	O	L	C	D	E	T	A	R	E	G	A	X	E	O
T	R	E	H	N	U	S	N	A	S	T	I	M	U	L	A	T	E	S	O
O	D	O	D	O	D	O	M	R	C	R	E	G	N	U	H	P	A	M	S
L	T	E	S	U	R	U	L	E	E	K	A	L	S	O	T	S	S	S	N
Y	E	H	M	S	C	T	C	A	L	D	S	N	E	H	T	E	E	I	R
N	N	A	E	A	E	E	S	E	T	B	O	L	O	O	K	C	L	E	E
A	O	H	V	R	L	R	T	L	S	N	O	M	E	M	A	N	G	E	C
M	I	A	I	I	E	B	T	O	E	W	E	R	W	E	T	A	G	T	N
P	T	V	N	Y	N	A	E	S	T	E	E	M	P	E	P	N	U	N	O
E	N	I	T	L	E	G	S	B	G	A	P	I	S	H	N	I	R	E	C
O	E	N	H	I	A	F	J	O	N	N	L	D	G	R	T	F	T	S	K
P	M	G	E	A	R	N	I	O	N	A	I	E	U	H	O	L	S	B	R
L	E	T	I	D	E	S	D	L	B	F	C	B	E	R	T	T	A	A	O
E	T	O	R	S	T	A	T	E	D	S	O	S	R	P	A	G	C	E	W
T	H	A	T	H	C	A	E	E	M	A	N	R	S	U	E	T	A	A	H
Y	E	H	T	D	A	Y	D	E	I	R	R	O	W	E	T	M	I	I	F
R	A	E	Y	L	S	U	O	D	N	E	M	E	R	T	R	S	I	O	N
D	E	K	N	I	L	N	A	C	Y	T	I	S	E	B	O	T	I	T	N
O	T	H	E	R	S	R	E	D	R	O	S	I	D	H	C	U	S	D	O
D	O	O	F	X	E	D	N	I	E	I	R	O	L	A	C	H	G	I	H

ENCIRCLE ANY WORD IN THE ABOVE PUZZLE WHICH IS SIMILAR TO ANY BELOW WORD:
1. DISTURBING STRESSORS REDUCE TOTAL SLEEP TIME, SHORT SLEEP DURATION INDUCES WEIGHT GAIN, AND STRESS CAN BE BLAMED TO BE THE REASON FOR LEAVING THE JOBS. MANY PEOPLE MENTION HAVING STRESS IN THEIR DAILY LIFE AND STATED THAT EACH DAY THEY ARE TREMENDOUSLY WORRIED, ALSO THE LACK OF SLEEP STIMULATES THE EXAGERATED HUNGER FOR HIGH-CALORIE INDEX FOOD
2. THEN OBESITY CAN BE LINKED TO STRESS AND MANY OTHER FACTORS AND DISORDERS SUCH AS "MENTAL HEALTH PROBLEMS, WORK ABSENTEEISM, FINANCES STRUGGLES, AND NEW MODERN CONCERNS"
3. EXTRA WORDS: LOOK, AT, MAP, TO, LET, SUN, DO, YEAR, SO, NAME, CLOCK

Word search Puzzle-Game D

T	O	F	E	Y	S	I	N	I	T	I	A	T	E	D	O	K	C	A	D
H	S	O	G	T	E	S	I	C	R	E	X	E	T	W	O	I	A	E	I
E	T	L	A	I	L	H	S	I	S	Y	L	A	R	A	P	D	N	S	A
O	R	A	T	V	F	I	T	F	E	R	U	L	I	A	F	N	C	I	B
N	E	C	R	I	Y	G	S	I	S	O	T	P	O	P	A	E	E	R	E
S	S	I	O	T	T	H	N	X	N	E	N	U	M	M	I	Y	R	S	T
E	S	S	H	C	I	S	O	D	O	B	L	O	O	D	Y	A	C	I	E
T	G	Y	S	A	S	E	I	T	I	V	I	T	C	A	R	T	L	S	S
R	N	H	L	N	N	D	T	O	T	S	S	S	Y	L	O	S	O	O	S
Y	I	P	E	I	E	E	A	B	A	I	E	T	T	U	T	I	T	R	E
O	W	S	E	M	T	N	C	E	V	G	L	O	O	N	A	S	T	E	L
B	O	E	P	O	N	T	I	S	I	N	U	R	K	G	M	O	I	L	B
E	L	I	A	T	I	A	L	I	T	A	C	M	I	I	M	T	N	C	I
S	L	T	N	I	D	R	P	T	C	L	E	H	N	N	A	A	G	S	S
I	O	I	D	V	E	Y	M	Y	A	L	L	O	E	J	L	M	S	O	R
T	F	V	R	A	C	B	O	B	N	I	O	P	S	U	F	O	E	I	E
Y	H	I	E	T	U	F	C	T	E	N	M	E	U	R	N	R	G	R	V
I	T	T	W	I	D	P	B	H	V	G	E	T	A	Y	I	E	A	E	E
S	I	C	O	O	E	E	F	A	I	N	D	U	C	E	O	H	M	T	R
O	W	A	L	N	R	R	M	T	R	H	C	I	H	W	R	T	A	R	R
A	S	S	O	C	I	A	T	E	D	R	I	V	E	N	P	A	D	A	I

ENCIRCLE ANY WORD IN THE ABOVE PUZZLE WHICH IS SIMILAR TO ANY BELOW WORD:

1. THE ONSET OF OBESITY IS ASSOCIATED WITH FOLLOWING ACTIVITIES:
   -PHYSICAL INACTIVITY, -SLEEP SHORTAGE, -RISE OF STRESS, -LOWER MOTIVATION AND REDUCED INTENSITY OF SELF-INITIATED PHYSICAL EXERCISE AND HIGH SEDENTARY ACTIVITIES
2. THE COMPLICATIONS OF OBESITY ARE DRIVEN BY: THE ACTIVATION OF PRO-INFLAMMATORY SIGNALLING MOLECULES THAT INDUCE CYTOKINE STORM WHICH CAUSE ATHEROMATOSIS, LUNG INJURY, APOPTOSIS, KIDNEY FAILURE, IMMUNE PARALYSIS, DIABETES TWO, CANCER, ARTERIOSCLEROSIS, BLOOD CLOTTING, AND IRREVERSIBLE DAMAGES
3. EXTRA WORDS: GET, LESS, BFM, TRY, TO, FIX, PFB, STAY, FIT, GO, OWE, HOPE

Word search Puzzle-Game E

C	U	F	S	O	F	T	H	R	E	E	B	M	I	A	B	O	V	E	A	M	F	B	S	S
O	L	I	R	P	R	E	V	E	N	T	E	A	O	V	E	R	W	E	I	G	H	T	I	N
N	T	G	O	R	I	S	K	A	I	O	V	E	R	E	A	T	I	N	G	B	R	O	M	S
S	I	H	I	S	O	L	U	T	I	O	N	S	H	I	G	H	C	C	E	E	S	B	M	E
U	M	T	V	F	I	F	T	Y	C	A	L	O	R	I	E	R	E	I	S	D	E	E	U	L
M	A	E	A	A	N	Y	O	N	E	C	A	N	B	E	E	V	N	S	N	I	C	S	N	B
P	T	R	H	H	E	A	L	E	R	H	A	V	E	A	I	G	F	E	S	I	R	I	E	A
T	E	K	E	E	P	S	A	C	T	I	O	N	S	T	F	U	O	T	H	A	T	T	S	T
I	M	F	B	P	L	A	N	W	E	E	K	E	C	L	L	Y	D	E	M	E	R	Y	E	E
O	R	D	A	Y	L	E	A	S	T	I	D	A	B	P	H	Y	S	I	C	A	L	L	Y	G
N	E	S	N	O	I	T	N	E	V	R	E	T	N	I	T	N	E	M	T	A	E	R	T	E
T	P	O	T	E	N	T	I	A	L	S	C	O	R	E	L	I	F	E	S	T	Y	L	E	V
I	H	B	S	A	B	E	M	O	T	I	V	A	T	E	D	F	I	X	G	O	A	L	S	T
O	F	I	V	E	C	O	N	D	I	T	I	O	N	S	Y	T	I	V	I	T	C	A	N	I
N	T	I	M	E	S	S	E	D	E	N	T	A	R	Y	M	O	N	I	T	O	R	S	N	U
O	R	E	K	N	I	R	D	H	U	N	D	R	E	D	A	T	G	N	I	C	U	D	E	R
T	S	T	O	P	D	O	S	E	C	I	O	H	C	H	E	A	L	T	H	Y	E	E	R	F
H	E	A	V	Y	P	R	O	M	O	T	E	R	L	O	R	T	N	O	C	F	L	E	S	O
D	I	E	T	L	A	U	D	I	V	I	D	N	I	E	H	T	E	M	P	O	W	E	R	O
F	O	R	E	T	A	L	U	G	E	R	F	L	E	S	D	E	T	E	R	M	I	N	E	D
D	E	S	O	P	X	E	N	O	U	T	C	O	M	E	D	U	L	C	N	I	A	N	D	C
M	O	R	E	L	A	C	S	E	T	U	N	I	M	A	N	A	G	E	S	A	H	O	H	W

ENCIRCLE ANY WORD IN THE ABOVE PUZZLE WHICH IS SIMILAR TO ANY BELOW WORD IN "QUOTES"

1. ENCIRCLE IN THE ABOVE PUZZLE "TWO CONDITIONS" EXPRESSED BY KEY WORDS STARTING WITH THE LETTER "O" THAT RELATE TO THE FOLLOWING HEALTHY RISK BEHAVIORS: "HRB": "REDUCING THE CONSUMPTION OF FRUIT/ VEGETABLES, INCREASED PHYSICAL INACTIVITY/ SEDENTARY BEHAVIOR, OVEREATING HIGH CALORIE FOOD, EXPOSED TO STRESSFUL CONDITIONS"
2. THEN "THE INDIVIDUAL SOLUTIONS" "TO REMEDY THE ABOVE CONDITIONS":
3. "LIFESTYLE TREATMENT INTERVENTIONS" TO EMPOWER THE INDIVIDUAL WHO HAS TO: "FIX GOALS AND PLAN THAT INCLUDE ULTIMATE ACTIONS, SELF-MANAGE; SELF-CONTROL; BE SELF-DETERMINED, BE-MOTIVATED TO SELF-REGULATE AND SELF MONITOR":
   -"WEIGHT": "AS BEING PHYSICALLY ACTIVE FOR AT LEAST ONE HUNDRED AND FIFTY MINUTES IN THE WEEK, STOP/PREVENT THE RISE OF WEIGHT AND KEEP A HEALTHY BMI
   -DIET: NOT A HEAVY DRINKER, EATING FRUIT/VEGETABLES FIVE OR MORE TIMES PER DAY AND HAVE AT LEAST A SCORE OF THREE" ON THE SCALE OF "HBS"
4. SUBSEQUENTLY "THE ULTIMATE OUTCOME OF THE TREATMENT IS: THAT ANYONE CAN BE A POTENTIAL HEALER/FIGHTER OF THE ABOVE CONDITIONS"
5. EXTRA WORDS: "IMMUNE, BFM"

www.ingramcontent.com/pod-product-compliance
Lightning Source LLC
Jackson TN
JSHW071722100425
82351JS00004B/7